Clinical Manual of
Pain Management
in Psychiatry

Clinical Manual of Pain Management in Psychiatry

Raphael J. Leo, M.D.
Associate Professor, State University of New York at Buffalo
School of Medicine and Biomedical Sciences;
Department of Psychiatry and
Center for Comprehensive Multidisciplinary Pain Management
Erie County Medical Center
Buffalo, New York

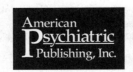

American Psychiatric Publishing, Inc.

Washington, DC
London, England

If you would like to buy between 25 and 99 copies of this or any other APPI title, you are eligible for a 20% discount; please contact APPI Customer Service at appi@psych.org or 800-368-5777. If you wish to buy 100 or more copies of the same title, please e-mail us at bulksales@psych.org for a price quote.

Copyright © 2007 American Psychiatric Publishing, Inc.
ALL RIGHTS RESERVED

Manufactured in the United States of America on acid-free paper
11   10   09   08   07   5   4   3   2   1
First Edition

Typeset in Adobe's Formata and AGaramond.

American Psychiatric Publishing, Inc.
1000 Wilson Boulevard, Arlington, VA 22209-3901
www.appi.org

Library of Congress Cataloging-in-Publication Data
Leo, Raphael J., 1962–
    Clinical manual of pain management in psychiatry / by Raphael J. Leo.—1st ed.
        p. ; cm.
    Includes bibliographical references and index.
    ISBN 978-1-58562-275-7 (pbk. : alk. paper)
    1. Pain—Treatment—Handbooks, manuals, etc. 2. Pain—Psychological aspects—Handbooks, manuals, etc. 3. Psychotherapy—Handbooks, manuals, etc. 4. Chronic pain—Handbooks, manuals, etc. I. Title.
    [DNLM: 1. Pain—therapy. 2. Chronic Disease—psychology. 3. Pain—psychology. WL 704 L576m 2007]
    RB127.L3966 2007
    616′.0472—dc22

                                                                          2007018819

British Library Cataloguing in Publication Data
A CIP record is available from the British Library.

Contents

List of Tables

List of Figures

Preface

The text of this manual, an update of the *Concise Guide to Pain Management for Psychiatrists,* was written in recognition of the significant advances in, and dynamism within, the field of pain medicine. Frequently, references are made to the importance of multidisciplinary, comprehensive treatment of the patient with pain. Nonetheless, the role of the psychiatrist and mental health practitioner in pain management continues to be the focus in this text. The contributory role of the psychiatrist in evaluation and assessment, pharmacologic management, psychotherapeutic interventions, and comprehensive treatment planning is emphasized. While interventional approaches to pain management are discussed herein, the importance of examining psychological variables that can limit outcomes and that may preclude undertaking aggressive, interventional approaches is elaborated on.

Information has been evolving regarding the biological substrates underlying both pain and psychiatric comorbidities (e.g., depression). Such knowledge expands the care and management of patients afflicted with pain and common psychiatric comorbidities. Particularly extensive revisions have been made in the sections describing the use of psychiatric and other adjunctive medications in pain management. While there is ample discussion of the role of opiates and weak analgesics in pain management, concerns frequently arise pertaining to long-term adverse effects, dependence, and behaviors resembling addiction (i.e., pseudoaddiction). Discussion of these issues has been expanded in the current edition. Effort is directed at delineating the utility of adjunctive treatments, including evolving data on the use of antidepressants and related medications, in the care of patients with chronic pain.

An overview of chronic pain conditions is presented, with an update of trends in treatment approaches that have been developed since publication of the Concise Guide edition. Finally, emerging legal and forensic issues pertinent to pain medicine have been updated in this text.

The positive comments that were received about the Concise Guide edition of the book were gratifying. It is this author's hope that the manual is still more useful to those psychiatrists and mental health practitioners who wish to devote their skills and expertise to the care of patients with pain.

Disclosure of competing interests: The author has no competing interests or conflicts to declare.

1

Introduction

Pain is one of the most ubiquitous health problems in the United States. Estimates suggest that 10%–20% of Americans have some form of chronic pain condition (Gatchel and Okifuji 2006). The impact of pain is far-reaching, adversely affecting vocational endeavors and contributing significantly to disability (Andersson 1999; White and Gordon 1982). The economic impact of chronic pain is enormous when one considers health care costs (estimated at over $70 billion annually) as well as the costs of absenteeism, reduced productivity, and disability compensation (estimated at over $150 billion annually) (Gatchel and Okifuji 2006). In addition, pain interferes with individuals' activities, interests, and relationships and limits the enjoyment of life.

Significant losses can accompany chronic pain (e.g., losses of income and autonomy). Patients may experience guilt, blaming themselves for their inability to overcome or master pain. In the home, the patient's role, and consequently the roles of others, may require modification, leading perhaps to strained relationships.

Pain is a common complaint among patients seeking medical attention. Despite the pervasiveness of pain and its multiple ramifications, the management of pain has often been elusive to clinicians. This is particularly true when

1

one considers the diversity of pain disorders that lack clear identifiable etiologies or when pain exceeds expectations given the underlying medical condition. Complex pain in a patient (i.e., pain that has not responded to common pain medications and interventions) can present an enormous burden to medical services.

Increasing attention has been directed to the issues of pain management, mobilized in part by the efforts of organizations that educate the public about pain management, such as the Compassion in Dying Federation, and by the standards of the Joint Commission on Accreditation of Healthcare Organizations (JCAHO). In addition, pain management has received increased attention from the medical community as a result of societal demands for more effective and comprehensive treatment. JCAHO requires that physicians consider pain as the fifth vital sign and that pain severity be documented by means of a standardized pain scale and be appropriately managed. Pain management also has received greater political and legal attention. Congress passed a provision, subsequently signed into law by President Clinton, declaring the decade 2001–2010 the "decade of pain control and research." From a medicolegal standpoint, physicians have been disciplined by state regulatory boards after review of medical records suggested negligence based on inadequate pain treatment (Albert 2001; Charatan 1999). Cumulatively, each of the aforementioned influences increases the external pressure, ensuring that physicians become current in effective pain management.

Origins and Development of Pain Management

Pain management first emerged as a subspecialty of anesthesiology. The need for the development of the science underlying pain and the skills for its treatment prompted efforts to refine training strategies and provide specialized pain clinics. Since the first pain clinic's appearance in 1951, approximately 3,800 pain clinics, programs, and solo practices have been established in the United States. This expansion points to the enormous need for specialized settings and specialists to work toward the amelioration of pain.

However, it became readily apparent that the knowledge and skills required of pain practitioners far exceeded those skills available to traditional anesthesiology training models. In addition to physical discomfort, patients with pain experience marked emotional distress. Emotional factors (e.g., depression and anxiety) not only emerge as a consequence of pain but also can contribute to pain, thereby exacerbating and maintaining it. Psychological factors can likewise interfere with treatment adherence and efficacy. Patients' frustration caused by ongoing pain, the effects on functioning, and the impact on families and relationships can contribute significantly to psychiatric morbidity. As a result of these factors, leaders in pain management training declared traditional medical models of pain to be too shortsighted and required a modification in traditional training conceptualizations (Loeser 2001).

Interdisciplinary Pain Medicine

Pain medicine has emerged as a medical subspecialty in its own right. Although not yet universally accepted, the term *pain medicine* is intended to encompass the principles of pain management and embody an interdisciplinary approach. Currently, specialists in pain medicine view pain as a distinct multifactorial illness (Gallagher 1999). Thus, no one discipline embodies the skills and mastery required to address pain. Rather, management and treatment of pain require the joint efforts of multiple clinical specialties, each of which can contribute to the effective treatment of pain. Hence, the skills of the anesthesiology expert can be complemented by the rehabilitation skills of the physiatrist and the psychotherapeutic and psychopharmacologic skills of the psychiatrist.

In 1998, the American Board of Psychiatry and Neurology (ABPN) and the American Board of Physical Medicine and Rehabilitation joined the American Board of Anesthesiology in recognizing pain management as an interdisciplinary subspecialty. Regardless of the primary discipline, pain medicine subspecialists need to understand the anatomy and physiology of pain perception, the psychological factors modifying the pain experience, and the basic principles of pain management.

Eligibility for the certifying examination in pain medicine requires that the applicant possess a medical license. The applicant must also be board certified in one of the aforementioned disciplines and, as of 2006, must have completed residency training in pain medicine approved by the Accreditation Council for Graduate Medical Education (ACGME).

Currently, the ACGME is refining fellowship training in pain medicine to reflect multiple disciplines. Toward this end, efforts are currently under way to specify the training experiences, didactics, and rotations in anesthesiology as well as psychiatry, neurology, and physical medicine and rehabilitation. Parameters for specialty tracks in pain medicine for each of these disciplines may also become available.

ABPN diplomates were first eligible to sit for the subspecialty certification examination in 2000. Subspecialty certification is appropriate for psychiatrists whose practices are largely devoted to pain management. However, given the pervasiveness of pain complaints, even the general psychiatrist will encounter pain management issues among his or her patients, and the general psychiatrist should also have the training and experience to recognize and treat basic psychiatric issues associated with pain. This book provides a concise guide to the psychiatric aspects of the management of pain.

Traditional Medical Models of Pain Management Versus the Current Biopsychosocial Paradigm

In traditional medical models of pain management, pain is seen as a signal of underlying disease or a pathophysiologic state. The physician is proactive in undertaking pharmacologic and other treatment interventions to treat the underlying disease state or relieve pain. The focus is on the disorder rather than on the person with the disorder. Consequently, the physician enlisted to treat the patient with pain first makes a determination as to the etiology of the pain. In ambiguous cases, there is often an exhaustive search for biomedical causes and treatment. When such efforts fail, the patient is dismissed as being "untreatable," and he or she is often left to persist in pain, with no improvement in functional adaptations.

In these traditional models there is a dualistic notion of pain, dividing it by organic versus psychogenic causes. Thus, there is a tendency to attribute to psychic factors any pain process in which the physical causes cannot be fully delineated. Similarly, if the pain complaints seem disproportionate to the underlying disease or if the pain fails to respond to treatment as expected, there is a belief that psychological processes underlie the pain. For many patients with chronic pain, such dualistic notions are inadequate (Boissevain and McCain 1991; Lynch 1992).

Frustrated by an inability to account for or to explain the cause of a patient's pain or by a feeling of futility or defeat when faced with a patient who persistently experiences pain despite the clinician's best efforts, the clinician may cease to take the patient's complaints seriously. For such patients, psychiatry becomes the treatment of last resort, prompted by resignation that the pain is psychic rather than somatic. Pain patients do not often think of themselves as needing to see a psychiatrist. Physicians are accustomed to hearing such patients ask, "Why do I have to see a psychiatrist?" The implication that the pain could be psychogenic can contribute to patients' distress. They may perceive that their doctors have given up on them, that their pain complaints are no longer taken seriously, or that they are being blamed for their persistent pain despite treatment (Gamsa 1994). (See Table 1–1 for a summary of the traditional pain model.)

Current conceptualizations of pain medicine adopt a biopsychosocial perspective (Engel 1977) (see Table 1–1). This model contends that the health status of individuals with chronic illnesses, the course of the illness, and the outcome of treatment are influenced by the interaction of biological, psychological, and social factors. The model provides a useful paradigm in which to view chronic pain states. The focus is on the rehabilitation and reclamation of the pain patient in the context of the pivotal doctor–patient relationship. Pain is viewed not exclusively as a signal of disease but as an experience with biological, psychological, and social derivatives. The treatment hinges on patient participation, and the physician serves as a guide, teacher, and interventionist to facilitate the rehabilitation process. The goal, therefore, is not necessarily a cure, because in many cases pain can be a chronic or even lifelong process. The biopsychosocial paradigm addresses relief from pain while addressing the impact of the pain condition on other aspects of one's functioning, relationships, vocational adaptations, and emotional well-being. The patient's emotional experiences, beliefs, and expectations can determine the outcome of treatment and are fully emphasized as the focus of treatment intervention. The biopsychosocial perspective pursues and examines psychological and social facets of the patient's pain experience without discounting the pain based on the presence of such facets. The goal is to identify and rectify any impediments to recovery and rehabilitation.

Role of Psychiatrists in Interdisciplinary Pain Medicine

Comprehensive pain treatment programs involving interdisciplinary, multimodal treatment approaches are often required in treating complex and dis-

Table 1–1. Traditional versus biopsychosocial models of pain

	Traditional pain model	Biopsychosocial model
View of pain	As an illness	As an experience
Determinants of pain	Disease	Biological, social, and psychological factors
Responsibility for treatment	Physician	Patient
Role of clinician	Expert on pain relief	Educator, motivator, physician-healer
Role of patient	Passive	Proactive
Goal(s) of treatment	Cure or pain relief	Increased function Improved quality of life Restored or improved relationships
Methods	Pharmacologic Technical	Educational Motivational Interpersonal Psychological Pharmacologic Technical
Focus of attention	Somatic complaints Pain as corresponding to pathology; if pain does not correspond, it is not real	Reciprocal relationship between somatic complaints and emotion, psychological processes, and interpersonal functions
	Disregard for patient's beliefs related to pain	Regard for patient's beliefs related to pain
	Focus on cause of pain	Focus on widespread impact of pain on life

abling pain conditions. Encompassing specialists in the fields of anesthesiology, neurology, psychiatry, psychology, and rehabilitation medicine, such programs are directed at implementing measures whereby the patient gains mastery over pain and refines cognitive styles and coping strategies (Jensen et al. 1994, 2001). Such comprehensive treatment programs are effective in producing symptomatic pain relief, reducing affective distress, and improving adaptive functioning and quality of life (Flor et al. 1992; Jensen et al. 2001; Skevington et al. 2001). The duration of effects appears to be sustained over time, reducing disability and health care utilization (Flor et al. 1992). Comprehensive pain treatment programs have emerged as the most efficacious and cost-effective means of addressing chronic pain, even among the most recalcitrant patients (Gatchel and Okifuji 2006).

Unfortunately, attrition rates can be quite high (Jensen et al. 1994). Factors predisposing to attrition include a long history of pretreatment pain, dependence on medications, multiple prior surgeries related to pain, and perceived lack of social support for maintaining participation in treatment (King and Snow 1989; Maruta et al. 1979).

Given that a significant number of psychosocial stressors and psychological comorbidities complicate the experience of chronic pain, there is wide acceptance of the necessity of psychiatric and other mental health practitioners in the comprehensive assessment and treatment of patients with pain. General psychiatric training renders the psychiatrist particularly well suited for the treatment of pain (Leo et al. 2003). Traditionally, psychiatrists view patients holistically and adopt a biopsychosocial perspective. Psychiatrists are trained in communication skills and are familiar with an array of pharmacologic agents that can reduce pain.

The psychiatrist enlisted to care for the pain patient can perform a variety of functions pivotal to the biopsychosocial approach (Table 1–2). Psychiatrists may choose the roles they wish to assume in pain treatment as defined by their skills, training, and expertise and by the collaborative efforts of other clinicians. Thus, psychiatrists might serve a role in diagnosing and managing discrete psychiatric disorders that accompany pain or interfere with treatment. Psychiatrists might be involved in facilitating the patient's adaptation after trauma or injury resulting in pain (e.g., motor vehicle crashes, work-related injuries), in interventions to treat pain (e.g., after an amputation), or in fostering improved quality of life, including social and vocational factors. Naturally, the psychiatrist can be in-

Table 1–2.   Role of psychiatrists in pain management
(biopsychosocial approach)

Assess pain.

Assess intervening variables that affect pain.

Prognosticate (consider factors that might influence pain, treatment compliance, and effects of treatment).

Determine problem areas for the patient.

Establish a treatment approach.

Delineate goals of treatment.

Reassess treatment efficacy.

Make modifications in the treatment plan as necessary.

volved in facilitating communication between the patient and clinicians with whom the patient interacts. (In some circumstances, the patient's perceptions of how he or she is being treated, believed, or construed may adversely affect therapeutic alliances and compromise the pain treatment team.)

Psychiatrists may be involved in the direct assessment and treatment of pain, in coordinating referrals to other pain specialists, and in all facets of the treatment plan. Conversely, they may respond to referrals from specialists in other disciplines to complement existing treatment strategies in which psychological factors are thought to be complicating recovery.

Psychiatrists can offer pharmacologic interventions for pain. They also can address emotional and cognitive sequelae of pain or its treatment and factors interfering with treatment (e.g., treatment adherence). The patient with chronic pain can become dependent on opiate analgesics, requiring psychiatric intervention. In some cases, the care of the pain patient may be entirely delegated to the psychiatrist.

Physicians seek psychiatric intervention to help in treating patients who have acute pain or painful terminal disorders, especially to address the psychological consequences and psychiatric comorbidities. More frequently, physicians seek consultation for patients with chronic pain with whom they are frustrated by lack of treatment response. Often, such patients are pejoratively labeled as noncompliant, uncooperative, attention seeking, medication seeking, or malingering (Gallagher 1999). Deciphering the relative contribution of biological and psychological variables to pain complaints requires evaluation by a psychiatrist with skills in the biopsychosocial assessment of pain. The patient's frustration caused by ongoing pain, the effects on functioning, and the impact on relationships contributes to significant psychiatric morbidity. It is not surprising, therefore, that the presence of chronic pain is a significant risk factor for suicide (Fishbain 1999). Thus, there is a great demand for psychiatrists to assist with pain management.

Key Points

- Pain is a ubiquitous health problem, the impact of which is far-reaching. On a societal level, the economic burdens are enormous. For the individual, pain adversely affects vocational endeavors, activities, interests, and relationships and limits enjoyment of life.
- From a biopsychosocial perspective, pain is viewed as an experience with biological, psychological, and social derivatives. This model provides a useful paradigm in which the focus is on bringing about rehabilitation of the pain patient and reclamation of his or her life, addressing symptomatic pain relief, reducing affective distress, improving adaptive functioning and quality of life, and thereby improving interpersonal and emotional well-being.
- Comprehensive pain treatment programs involving interdisciplinary, multimodal treatment approaches are often required for complex and disabling pain conditions.
- Interdisciplinary treatment programs involve the coordination and collaborative endeavors of a number of health care providers, with the goals of alleviating symptoms, enhancing patient independence, improving functional adaptation, addressing the psychological comorbidities accompanying pain, and improving psychosocial functioning.
- Within the biopsychosocial perspective, there are several pivotal roles that the psychiatrist can perform in the assessment, treatment, and ongoing management of the patient with pain.

References

Albert T: Doctor guilty of elder abuse for undertreating pain. Am Med News, July 23, 2001, pp 1, 4

Andersson GBJ: Epidemiological features of chronic low-back pain. Lancet 354:581–585, 1999

Boissevain MD, McCain GA: Toward an integrated understanding of fibromyalgia syndrome, I: medical and pathophysiologic aspects. Pain 45:227–238, 1991

Charatan F: Doctor disciplined for "grossly undertreating" pain. BMJ 319:728, 1999

Engel GL: The need for a new medical model: a challenge for biomedicine. Science 196:129–136, 1977

Fishbain DA: The association of chronic pain and suicide. Semin Clin Neuropsychiatry 4:221–227, 1999

Flor H, Fydrich T, Turk DC: Efficacy of multidisciplinary pain treatment centers: a meta-analytic review. Pain 49:221–230, 1992

Gallagher RM: Treatment planning in pain medicine: integrating medical, physical and behavioral therapies. Med Clin North Am 83:823–849, 1999

Gamsa A: The role of psychological factors in chronic pain, II: a critical appraisal. Pain 57:17–29, 1994

Gatchel RJ, Okifuji A: Evidence-based scientific data documenting the treatment and cost-effectiveness of comprehensive pain programs for chronic nonmalignant pain. J Pain 7:779–793, 2006

Jensen MP, Turner JA, Romano JM: Correlates of improvement in multidisciplinary treatment of chronic pain. J Consult Clin Psychol 62:172–179, 1994

Jensen MP, Turner JA, Romano JM: Changes in beliefs, catastrophizing, and coping are associated with improvement in multidisciplinary pain treatment. J Consult Clin Psychol 69:655–662, 2001

King SA, Snow BR: Factors for predicting premature termination from a multidisciplinary inpatient chronic pain program. Pain 39:281–287, 1989

Leo RJ, Pristach CA, Streltzer J: Incorporating pain management training into the psychiatry residency curriculum. Acad Psychiatry 27:1–11, 2003

Loeser JD: Multidisciplinary pain programs, in Bonica's Management of Pain, 5th Edition. Edited by Loeser JD, Butler SH, Chapman CR, et al. Philadelphia, PA, Lippincott Williams & Wilkins, 2001, pp 255–264

Lynch M: Psychological aspects of reflex sympathetic dystrophy: a review of the adult and pediatric literature. Pain 49:337–347, 1992

Maruta T, Swanson DW, Swenson WM: Chronic pain: which patients may a pain-management program help? Pain 7:321–329, 1979

Skevington SM, Carse MS, Williams AC: Validation of the WHOQOL-100: pain management improves quality of life for chronic pain patients. Clin J Pain 17:264–275, 2001

White AA 3rd, Gordon SL: Synopsis: workshop on idiopathic low-back pain. Spine 7:141–149, 1982

2

Sensory Pathways of Pain and Acute Versus Chronic Pain

Pain is a multidimensional concept (Loeser 1982), with biological, psychological, and social components (Figure 2–1). First, there is a sensory component of the pain experience—an unpleasant sensation detected in the body and processed in the central nervous system (CNS). This process, referred to as *nociception*, relies on the transfer of information about the sensory experience from receptors in the periphery through nerves to the spinal cord and on to the brain.

Second, there is an assessment of the unpleasant sensory experience. This assessment involves a cognitive awareness of the sensation arising from the periphery that the person labels as pain. Not all sensations are painful; some can be construed as unusual, uncomfortable, or irritating but not painful. Thus, the common pins-and-needles sensation in one's foot might be described as the foot "falling asleep" but not as pain. Similarly, one may experience an itch, a twitch, or other noxious sensations (e.g., burning, throbbing) that are labeled as painful.

Third, there is a perception and cognitive appraisal that the discomfort is associated with suffering. This subsumes not only the sensation and awareness

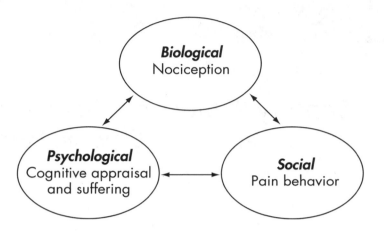

Figure 2–1.   Dimensions of pain and the biopsychosocial model.

of pain but also the reactions to the experience (e.g., distress, dysphoria, anxiety, hopelessness). The experience of pain may connote various experiences for the individual, including many unpleasant emotional states.

The final dimension of pain consists of the pain behaviors displayed by the patient in response to the unpleasant experience. Here the person conveys to others how much distress he or she is experiencing. These behaviors can be verbal (e.g., "Wow, this really hurts!"), paraverbal (e.g., moaning), or nonverbal (e.g., guarding an affected limb, splinting, wearing a neck brace, taking medication, reclining).

The neurophysiologic substrates of the pain experience are discussed in this chapter. The first part of the chapter comprises a discussion of the sensory pathways and mechanisms. The second part focuses on distinctions between acute and chronic pain.

Pain-Relaying Pathways and Mechanisms

In their most basic aspects, the pain relay pathways involve three sets of neurons. First-order neurons relay noxious information from the periphery or viscera to the spinal cord. Second-order neurons relay sensory information from the spinal cord to the thalamus. Third-order neurons arising from the thalamus send information to higher brain regions where complex processing of the pain experience occurs.

First-Order Neurons: Relay to the Spinal Cord

The detection of pain requires that information regarding injury, trauma, and noxious stimulation be detected by a transducer. Transducers serve the purpose of taking information (e.g., changes in temperature, chemical irritation, pressure) from some location on the body surface, muscles, or internal organs and converting it into neurochemical information that is interpretable by the brain. The transducers for pain include the free nerve endings of the first-order neurons in the pain pathway (i.e., the Aδ and C neurons). These neurons have long dendrites with fine terminal arborizations present in the skin, muscle, connective tissue, joints, bone, and internal organs. When these neurons are stimulated, action potentials extend from the dendrites to the cell body (in the dorsal root ganglion) and from the axon to the spinal cord.

Information relayed about other nonnoxious sensory modalities (e.g., pressure, touch, proprioception) is detected by other types of sensory transducers. These include pacinian corpuscles, Meissner's corpuscles, and other transducers. When sufficiently stimulated, these receptors in turn pass information along another set of first-order neurons, the Aβ neurons.

First-order neurons differ in their diameter, myelination, and, therefore, electrical conduction rates (Table 2–1). Miscalculating the intended alignment of a hammer to the intended target (i.e., the head of the nail), one can quickly appreciate the pain relay process once the swift blow of the hammer makes inadvertent contact with the fingers of the hand holding the nail in place. First, Aβ fibers, responding to low-threshold touch receptors, relay information about the blunt object making contact with the hand. Simultaneously (when the stimulus is disconcertingly high, as in this example), high-threshold mechanoreceptors and heat receptors are activated. This information is conducted quickly and robustly, via Aδ fibers, immediately after the injury. Aδ fiber information is well localized, sharp, pricking, and pulsating but very short-lived. Shortly thereafter, C fibers relay information from the injured hand—information that is less definitive or localized than that of the Aδ fibers (Besson and Chaouch 1987). These C fibers mediate the slowly emerging, more

Table 2–1.   Sensory neural fiber types of first-order neurons

	Aβ	Aδ	C
Diameter	Large (5–15 μm)	Intermediate (1–4 μm)	Thin (0.5–1.5 μm)
Myelination	Yes	Yes	No
Conduction rate	Fast (30–70 m/s)	Fast (12–30 m/s)	Slow (0.5–2.0 m/s)
Sensory information	Cutaneous touch and pressure	Well localized Sharp pain	Poorly localized Dull, aching pain

persistent, dull, aching, and burning pain that is experienced. All three types of fibers relay information to the dorsal horn of the spinal cord, where they synapse directly, or indirectly through interneurons, on the second-order neurons involved in the nociceptive pathway (Byers and Bonica 2001).

Viscera are also supplied by C fibers and Aδ fibers. These are activated by inflammatory processes, ischemia, disease, rapid distention, and contraction. These events trigger free nerve endings to transduce the noxious information into electrical information that is eventually transmitted to the dorsal horn.

Pain from the face is relayed to the CNS through the fifth cranial (i.e., the trigeminal) nerve. Noxious information from the face is relayed via dendrites of one of the three branches of the trigeminal nerve, passes through to the trigeminal ganglion (containing the cell bodies of the trigeminal nerves), and passes to the second-order neurons in the pons and medulla. In a pattern that parallels that of spinal cord pathways, information is ultimately relayed to the thalamus and higher brain structures (Dubner and Bennett 1983). The face and mouth have a high density of pain transducers and pain fibers and are thus exquisitely sensitive to stimulation. Similarly, the representation of the face and mouth in the somatosensory cortex of the brain is extensive, suggesting that processing and encoding of sensory information from the face and mouth is quite elaborate.

Dorsal Horn Anatomy

The gray matter of the spinal cord is classified by histological characteristics into 10 layers or laminae (referred to as *Rexed layers*). The dorsal horn contains 6 of these. Those layers that are essential in the pain processing pathways include laminae I, II, and V, primarily where Aδ and C fibers terminate (Terman and Bonica 2001). Cells within the dorsal horn include those that are nociceptive specific (i.e., respond to noxious stimulation). Other cells respond only to innocuous stimuli, whereas still others, referred to as *wide dynamic range* (WDR) cells, respond to noxious and innocuous stimuli but discharge at a higher frequency to noxious stimuli.

The substantia gelatinosa, contained within lamina II, has a significant role in modulating pain. This substance involves small interneurons that serve as control switches or gates through which sensory information from the periphery is either enhanced or depressed. Certain of these interneurons (i.e., islet cells) are inhibitory, whereas others (i.e., stalked cells) are excitatory. The substantia gelatinosa receives extensive serotonergic and noradrenergic input from nerve fibers emanating from higher brain centers, which likewise influences the gating process.

When one experiences pain from a joint, massage of the overlying skin may reduce some of that discomfort. This phenomenon, referred to as *counterirritation,* is attributed to the gating mechanism of the substantia gelatinosa. Massaging, by stimulating the tactile receptors of the skin, activates Aβ fibers. These fibers in turn activate interneurons within the substantia gelatinosa that serve to inhibit pain-mediating pathways (Melzack and Wall 1965; Wall 1980). Counterirritation has been offered as an explanation to account for why certain therapeutic modalities can be effective in mitigating pain—for example, use of liniment or transcutaneous electrical nerve stimulation units.

Lamina V contains WDR cells with large receptive fields (i.e., they receive extensive inputs from multiple sources). For example, Aδ and C fibers arising from visceral structures enter lamina V. The WDR cells receiving the neural input from visceral organs simultaneously receive input from other sites. This process is the basis for referred pain (i.e., the interpretation of unpleasant sensory input arising from viscera as emanating from peripheral sites) (Pomeranz et al. 1968). Thus, hypoxic injury to the heart is perceived as pain in the left arm, because the afferents from the heart synapse on those lamina V cells of the left lower cervical and upper thoracic segments. The brain interprets the stimulation of those cells as pain originating in the left upper chest and arm.

Second-Order Neurons: The Spinothalamic Tract

The axons arising from neurons making up the spinothalamic tract emanate from the entire gray matter of the spinal cord. Most of these fibers cross to the other side of the spinal cord through the ventral commissure in the midline and ascend in the anterolateral aspect of the white matter (myelinated) portion of the spinal column. These fibers ascend without interruption through the spinal column and brain stem and terminate in the contralateral thalamus (Besson and Chaouch 1987; Dennis and Melzack 1977). However, a small number of fibers project to the ipsilateral thalamus. These pain relay pathways diverge into the two pathways within the spinothalamic system: the neo-spinothalamic (sensory-discriminative) and the paleospinothalamic (affective-motivational) pathways (Figure 2–2). The latter is considered to be a phylo-genetically older pathway.

Third-Order Neurons: The Thalamus and Beyond

The thalamus is the primary relay station for sensory information from the spinal cord to the cortex (Chudler and Bonica 2001; Rome and Rome 2000). The second-order neurons from the neospinothalamic tract terminate in the lateral aspect of the ventral posterior nucleus (VPN). Third-order neurons from the VPN relay information to the somatosensory cortex (parietal lobe). Through this pathway, discriminative aspects of pain, localization of the pain, and coordinated motor responses to the pain are possible (Rome and Rome 2000).

Information is relayed simultaneously from the paleospinothalamic path-way through a parallel pathway to the reticular formation, medial thalamus, hypothalamus, and prefrontal cortex (Giesler et al. 1994). The nociceptive system thereby influences affect, attention, cognition, and memory that relate to painful sensory information (Chudler and Bonica 2001). A stress reaction develops to noxious sensation, involving the hypothalamic-pituitary axis and autonomic nervous system (Giesler et al. 1994). Ultimately, this information is relayed to both cortices. As a result, the affective quality and coloring of the pain experience are possible. In addition, affective influences mediated by lim-bic involvement are likely to modulate pain. Thus, one's surprise (e.g., "I can't believe I hit my hand with the hammer!"), alarm (e.g., "I didn't see that com-ing!"), anger (e.g., "That was so stupid!"—along with use of expletives), and fear (e.g., "My hand is damaged for good!") are likely to shape the experience of pain. Mood states (e.g., a predisposition to anxiety or depression) can shape the cognitive strategies one employs to deal with the pain, one's sense of effi-cacy in dealing with the injury, and one's expectations for the future. The relay of pain information to the bilateral cortices adds a cognitive component to the

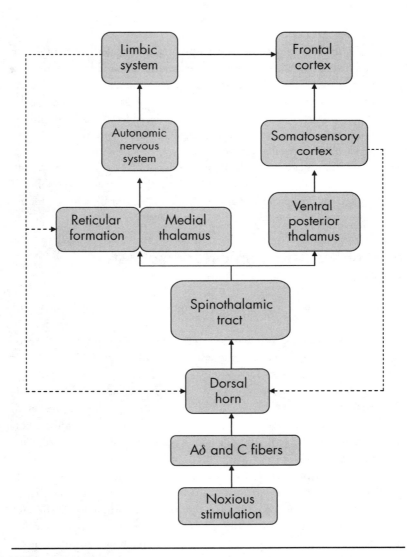

Figure 2–2. The affective-motivational pathway *(left)* and the sensory-discriminative pathway *(right).*

Note. Dashed line = inhibitory pathways; solid line = pain-facilitating pathways.

pain experience. Thus, the mutual influences of mood, cognition, expectation, and pain are mediated.

The frontal cortex mediates the cognitive processes underlying pain. These processes involve the identification and evaluation of, and decision making pertaining to, the noxious sensory information input from the periphery. Hence, immediate short-term problem solving can be undertaken (e.g., ignoring the hammering, preferring instead to tend to the injured hand). Other cognitive processes—such as one's expectations along with the attributions, beliefs, and meanings ascribed to the painful experience—are likewise derived from cortical processes and influence both the pain experience and the decision making around the pain. In addition, memory of the painful experience is established and encoded for further referral and to guide subsequent behaviors—for example, how (and whether) one tries carpentry again.

Role of the Autonomic Nervous System in Pain

The autonomic nervous system plays a significant role in pain. Signals of threat and danger are relayed to the hypothalamus. From there, specifically the posterior portion, information is relayed to the spinal cord (i.e., the thoracic and lumbar regions) by sympathetic neural pathways (McMahon 1991). Ultimately, fibers from the thoracolumbar regions innervate a number of endorgans producing activation (i.e., a state of heightened arousal). Those endorgan activities that are necessary for fight-or-flight responses are promoted, whereas those that are not necessary are suppressed. Thus, the information signaling threat or danger results in elevated heart rate and blood pressure, increased oxygen use, sweating, dilation of pupils, and increased glycogen utilization within muscles. Other organ functions (e.g., peristalsis) are inhibited.

The effects of sympathetic nervous system activity are relatively brief in duration because of the rapid release and degradation of norepinephrine and acetylcholine released in the mediation of the fight-or-flight response. More sustained reactions to stressors or threat are mediated by neuroendocrine effects, a product of adrenal medulla activation. Sympathetic nervous system activation of the adrenal gland results in release of norepinephrine and epinephrine, mimicking sympathetic activity.

Pain-Modulating Processes Within the Nervous System

The pain transmission pathways that have been presented thus far are simplistic. In reality, a number of processes can influence pain transmission from the periphery through the entire CNS. These mechanisms involve complex and dynamic interactions among various neurotransmitters, their receptors, and other pain-reducing and pain-augmenting processes. These are discussed briefly in the following sections.

Neurochemicals in Pain Processing

A number of neurotransmitters and chemical substrates are involved in pain transmission; several are listed in Table 2–2. For example, in the periphery, tissue injury results in the activation of a number of cellular processes that release chemical compounds that can activate free nerve endings for pain transmission (Snyder 1980), such as acetylcholine, bradykinin, histamine, potassium ion, and serotonin (Levine et al. 1993). Additional agents that are active within the CNS are also listed in Table 2–2. Some of these substances have a pain-promoting role, whereas others have a pain inhibitory role. Many of these substances are the targets of influence when analgesics are employed (e.g., anti-inflammatory agents and antidepressants), as is described further in Chapter 5, "Pharmacology of Pain," of this book.

Endogenous Opiates

The endogenous opiates consist of β-endorphin, enkephalins, and dynorphins (Sewell and Lee 1980). These are abundantly distributed throughout the CNS, thereby modulating pain transmission. Enkephalins are endogenous opiates found in the interneurons of the substantia gelatinosa that mediate the effects of inhibitory interneurons within the dorsal horn. Binding to opioid receptors, enkephalins can inhibit the release of substance P from nociceptors. In fact, intraspinal application of opiates (e.g., morphine) is thought to influence the enkephalin receptors, thereby mitigating pain transmission from the spinal cord. Cells producing β-endorphin arise from the hypothalamus and are thought to exert their influence within the limbic system and midbrain.

Table 2–2.   Mediators of pain processing and transmission

	Pain promoting	Pain inhibiting
Peripheral nervous system	Acetylcholine Adenosine Bradykinin Cytokines Glutamate Histamine K^+ Prostaglandins (E series) Serotonin Substance P	Endogenous opiates
Central nervous system	Cholecystokinin Glutamate Serotonin Norepinephrine Substance P	Endogenous opiates β-Endorphin Endorphins Dynorphins Serotonin Norepinephrine Neurotensin

Source.   Adapted from Terman GW, Bonica JJ: "Spinal Mechanisms and Their Modulation," in *Bonica's Management of Pain,* 3rd Edition. Edited by Loeser JD, Butler SH, Chapman CR, et al. Philadelphia, PA, Lippincott Williams & Wilkins, 2001, pp. 73–152.

Pain-Reducing Pathways

Several structures serve to diminish the pain sensory information coming into the CNS. Intuitively, pain-modulating mechanisms prevent the organism from being overcome by unbridled pain, thereby allowing the organism an opportunity to "escape" and tend to the injury. The four regions in the CNS that can function to reduce pain sensation and control pain awareness are 1) the cortex and limbic structures, 2) the midbrain (the periaqueductal gray [PAG]), 3) the rostral ventromedial medulla (RVM), and 4) the spinal dorsal horn (Besson and Chaouch 1987; Terman and Bonica 2001). The gating mechanism of the substantia gelatinosa within the dorsal horn was described earlier in this chapter. The cortex and reticular formation can influence attention, arousal, expectations of pain, and psychological factors that can in turn influence pain experiences. The specific mechanisms by which these structures influence pain have yet to be clarified.

The PAG is a midbrain structure with an abundance of opiate receptors. Neural connections extend from the PAG to neighboring serotonergic structures (e.g., the RVM) and noradrenergic structures (e.g., the dorsolateral ponto-mesencephalic tegmentum [DLPT]). The pain-modulating influences of the PAG are conducted predominately, if not exclusively, through the RVM. The RVM in turn projects onto the cells of the dorsal horn in laminae I, II, and V (Terman and Bonica 2001). Analgesia results if morphine is injected into the PAG, RVM, or amygdala. In μ-opiate receptor–deficient mice, morphine injection into the PAG, RVM, and amygdala is completely ineffective in mitigating pain. The μ-receptor, therefore, is responsible for the supraspinal analgesia produced by opiates, mediated through the PAG and RVM.

Additionally, axons of supraspinal nuclei extend down the spinal cord, synapse within the dorsal horn, and release monoamines that influence pain transmission (see Table 2–3). Essentially all of the serotonin-containing neurons in the dorsal horn originate from the RVM and the raphe nuclei. Thus, for example, stimulation of the RVM evokes serotonin release with resultant analgesia, an effect that can be blocked by concomitant serotonin antagonist (e.g., methysergide) administration. The analgesic effects of serotonin are thought to be mediated largely by 5-HT_{1A} receptors (Terman and Bonica 2001).

As with serotonin, norepinephrine released by axons extending from the locus coeruleus and DLPT and terminating within the dorsal horn can inhibit pain transmission (see Table 2–3). The analgesic effect of norepinephrine is thought to be mediated by activity at the α_2-receptor. Support for this is suggested by the fact that α_2-receptor agonists (e.g., clonidine) can produce analgesia. In addition, norepinephrine appears to be essential for opioid-induced analgesia; blockade of norepinephrine (e.g., by phentolamine) reduces the effects of systemically applied opioids. However, serotonin and norepinephrine have both nociceptive and antinociceptive effects depending on the specific receptor subtypes and the neural circuitry activated (see Table 2–3).

Opiate Receptors and Descending Inhibition of Pain Pathways

There are four classes of opiate receptors recognized to date (Terenius 1985). The μ-receptor is responsible for supraspinal analgesia. It also produces eu-

Table 2–3.   Monoamine neurotransmission involved in descending pain inhibition

		Effect on pain transmission	
Neurotransmitter and sources	Receptors	Inhibitory	Promoting
Serotonin	5-HT$_{1A}$	+	
Rostral ventromedial medulla	5-HT$_2$		+
Raphe nuclei	5-HT$_{1B}$	+	+
	5-HT$_3$	+	+
Norepinephrine	α_2	+	
Locus coeruleus	α_1		+
DLPT			

Note.   Serotonin and norepinephrine have both nociceptive (pain promoting) and antinociceptive (pain inhibiting) effects depending on the specific receptor subtypes and the neural circuitry activated. DLPT = dorsolateral pontomesencephalic tegmentum.
Source.   Adapted from Terman GW, Bonica JJ: "Spinal Mechanisms and Their Modulation," in *Bonica's Management of Pain,* 3rd Edition. Edited by Loeser JD, Butler SH, Chapman CR, et al. Philadelphia, PA, Lippincott Williams & Wilkins, 2001, pp. 73–152.

phoria from opiate use and is responsible for physical dependence. Physical effects of opiates (e.g., hypotension, decreased respirations, hypothermia, pruritus, and decreased gastrointestinal motility) are all attributed to μ-receptor activation from opiate use.

Analgesia on a spinal level is a result of the opiate activation of the κ-receptor. Activation results in pupil constriction and sedation. The δ-receptors also produce analgesia and are activated by endogenous opiates. The role of the σ-receptor is more controversial. It produces no analgesia but is responsible for the dysphoria, and possibly hallucinations, associated with opiate use. Because of these disparate effects, compared with other opiate receptors, there is controversy about whether the σ-receptor is actually an opiate receptor.

The μ-receptor produces more analgesia than the other types of receptors. It is also responsible for changes in respiratory activity, gastrointestinal motility, and sphincter tone produced by opiates. The μ-receptor is abundantly present in the dorsal horn, medulla, and the PAG. It is also responsible for pain modulation at peripheral nerve endings. Its abundance in the myenteric plexus is likely responsible for the effects of the opiates on gastrointestinal motility and sphincter tone.

Table 2–4.   Causes of chronic pain

Ongoing activation of pain pathways from the periphery can cause pain
to become chronic.

Peripheral nerves may be dysfunctional.

Motor reflexes may potentiate pain.

Dorsal horn can become sensitized.

Sympathetic nervous system can become a major contributor to
ongoing pain.

Cortical and limbic activity can contribute to pain.

Pain-Augmenting Mechanisms and the Emergence of Chronic Pain

When acute pain is inadequately treated, there is an increased risk of emergence of chronic pain. Several mechanisms are postulated to play a role in the development of chronic and enduring pain (see Table 2–4).

Ongoing abnormalities in peripheral tissues, with resultant inflammation, can result in activation of nociceptive pathways, rendering pain chronic. In such cases, treatment is best directed at the inflammatory mechanisms (e.g., aspirin or nonsteroidal anti-inflammatory agents). Peripheral nerves may become dysfunctional due to injury or disease (e.g., diabetes, infection, toxin exposure). Damaged neurons may fire spontaneously. Nociceptive fibers firing in this way are perceived in the CNS as signaling pain, yet in the peripheral tissues there may be no current injury. In such cases, antidepressants and anticonvulsants might be the most helpful treatment.

Trauma and injury can produce reflex motor activity in the vicinity of the injury, producing spasm. This process may initially serve a protective function in acute pain states, but in chronic pain states it can lead to aggravated muscle tension that exacerbates painful states (Zimmerman 1979).

The dorsal horn can become sensitized by a number of mechanisms that can potentiate chronic pain. Changes that occur within the dorsal horn may account for the maintenance of pain sensation that loses its relevance in its ability to signal danger. This sensitization appears to be related to changes mediated by CNS neurotransmitters, especially the excitatory neurotransmitter glutamate. With repeated stimulation (e.g., in poorly treated acute pain or in re-injury), glutamate activity can expand to include other receptors, including *N*-methyl-D-aspartate (NMDA) receptors. With expansion of glutamate activity, a series of intracellular processes occur that result in the heightened activation of dorsal horn cells, referred to as *wind up*. Such processes become difficult to interrupt from a therapeutic standpoint; however, NMDA receptor blockers (e.g., ketamine) can be helpful.

Ongoing NMDA activation can result in cell death. Death of neurons leaves areas of deafferentation in the spinal cord pathways. As a result, nearby sensory neurons often sprout collaterals into the deafferentated area to replace the synaptic connections lost after cell death. This replacement results in an innervation of pain pathways that correspond to the injured areas stimulated or activated by nearby undamaged areas.

The sympathetic nervous system can become a major contributor to ongoing pain (Zimmerman 1979). Trauma and injury trigger a sympathetic response that can effectively alter the neurochemical milieu of nociceptors in the periphery, along with causing changes in the microcirculation. This situation can alter the sensitivity of peripheral pain receptors, thereby augmenting pain sensitivity.

Pain can be maintained—despite lack of injury or even after effective healing—by the actions of the sympathetic nervous system. In such cases, protracted painful conditions can arise, such as reflex sympathetic dystrophy and complex regional pain disorder. Some of these disorders can be alleviated by blockade of sympathetic activity (i.e., sympatholysis); however, not all respond to sympatholytic techniques. Treatment for such disorders can include nerve blocks, sympathetic nerve blocks, and psychotropic medications (e.g., antidepressants and anticonvulsants).

Commensurate alterations in the thalamus and somatosensory cortex can occur after peripheral nerve injury. Thus, even after an amputation, the area of the somatosensory cortex corresponding to the amputated limb increases. Other cortical and limbic events can contribute to pain. The experience of pain can be shaped and influenced by the diffuse interconnections of the pain pathways with limbic and cortical pathways. In such cases, psychoactive medications, psychotherapy, and adjunctive therapeutic approaches such as relaxation training may be helpful modes of treatment.

Acute Versus Chronic Pain

The sensation of pain serves an adaptive function. Specifically, nociceptive pathways serve to alarm the organism that some damage or injury has been sustained and that efforts may need to be directed at tending to the injury and avoiding further injury. Consider a disorder such as Hansen's disease, also known as leprosy, which is characterized by dysfunction in pain-mediating pathways. Persons infected with *Mycobacterium leprae,* the agent that causes the disease, have deficits in pain perception. On the surface, this seems quite desirable; however, over the course of the illness, these patients sustain marked deficits in self-care and are exposed to hazards brought on by physical injury and infection. Death can result from the lack of appropriate awareness of the bodily warning mechanisms that would otherwise motivate treatment.

Problems arise when pain takes on a life of its own. Certainly, in medical conditions in which there is ongoing tissue damage—arthritis, for example—pain may likewise be ongoing. One might question the utility of such pain, because one certainly is aware of the trauma that warrants medical attention. On the other hand, and perhaps more troubling, there are situations in which pain persists despite healing (e.g., postherpetic neuralgia) or situations in which pathologic processes emerge within the CNS or the peripheral nervous system (or both) to produce aberrant activity that is interpreted and experienced as pain, as in Dejerine-Roussy syndrome (a pain syndrome related to thalamic stroke).

Classifications of Acute and Chronic Pain

Pain is classified in several ways, including the familiar categories of acute and chronic. For example, pain can be classified based on its temporal aspects, its etiology and its associated features from differing sources, and its functional significance (see Table 2–5). *Acute pain* has been customarily defined as pain that is less than 6 months in duration. *Chronic pain* is defined as pain persisting beyond 6 months (Crue 1983). There are always problems with arbitrary definitions such as these. For example, it becomes difficult to classify some painful conditions (e.g., migraine or osteoarthritis) based on temporal aspects. Migraine is a recurrent painful disorder that can persist for years, but the specific episodes of pain are relatively short-lived. Osteoarthritis, on the other hand,

Table 2–5.   Features distinguishing acute and chronic pain

	Acute pain	Chronic pain
Duration	<6 months	>6 months
Cause	Tissue damage, injury, inflammation	Pathophysiologic processes in the peripheral or CNS pathways Psychogenic factors
Biological utility	Yes	No
Psychological factors contributing	No	Yes

Note.   CNS = central nervous system.

is a chronic, progressive medical condition that is accompanied by a mixture of acute and chronic pain components. Acute pain can be precipitated by new injury, whereas chronic pain features can arise from prior injuries and sensitization of peripheral nervous system involvement.

Generally, acute pain is considered to be pain that serves self-protective functions. The value of the alarm functions of pain brought on by the inadvertent slamming of one's thumb with a hammer is obvious. Such pain, it is hoped, is discrete and mobilizes the person to take measures to minimize pain and prevent further injury. Conversely, chronic pain is considered to have lost such meaningful aspects. One is hard-pressed to arrive at any adaptive function gleaned from chronic neuropathic pains or fibromyalgia.

Acute pain arises from tissue injury, trauma, or inflammation. Chronic pain extends beyond the period of healing and can be brought on by pathophysiologic processes within the nervous system. Some pain states can be mediated by the ongoing barrage of peripheral pain sensors (i.e., nociceptors). The pathologic firing of peripheral or CNS pathways that mediate pain can also trigger chronic pain.

Another distinction between acute and chronic pain states is based on the presence of psychological and psychiatric conditions that accompany or aggravate the pain. The pain brought on by fracture or another traumatic injury is not necessarily accompanied by the personality changes and psychiatric disturbances that can accompany chronic pain states. Psychological sequelae of acute pain are likely to be discrete and obvious.

The long duration and pervasive effects of chronic pain states likely have an impact on a person's functioning. Naturally, pain can have profound effects on social, interpersonal, and emotional functioning. By virtue of the long-term course, there may be changes in mood, thought patterns, perceptions, and personality that accompany the pain. One's life experiences and ability to adapt to ongoing demands and stress are affected. Therefore, it is incomprehensible to address chronic pain without considering psychological and social functioning.

Categories of Chronic Pain

Chronic pain has been categorized as nociceptive, neuropathic, or psychogenic (Table 2–6). These classifications differ with respect to their characteristics and responsiveness to varying types of treatment interventions (Leo and Singh 2002; Portenoy 1989). For example, nociceptive pain responds to anti-inflammatory agents and opiate analgesics, whereas neuropathic pain responds to antidepressants, anticonvulsants, and opiates.

"Patienthood" as a Psychosocial State: The Patient With Simple Versus Chronic Pain

An array of factors can become central to the life experiences of the patient with chronic pain (Table 2–7). As a result of these factors, a number of emotional and psychological sequelae are associated with the chronic pain state. Physicians have long noted a puzzling discrepancy between physical disease status and progression and the patient's subjective experiences (Weisberg and Clavel 1999). Some patients with severe disease present few complaints and report less disability and emotional distress. Yet some others with little documented disease report severe symptoms and experience marked distress and disability.

Despite the pervasiveness of chronic pain, most individuals with chronic pain can nonetheless maintain basic functioning, work, and interests. They are able to work with their clinicians and other care providers and can respond with some relief to medications or interventions. At times, psychotherapeutic interventions may be required to address mood disturbances, stress, and coping. This cluster of patients is sometimes referred to as having simple chronic pain. Small proportions of patients with chronic pain are entirely debilitated by the pain and are sometimes referred to as having complex chronic pain (see

Table 2–6.   Categories of chronic pain

	Source	Localization	Features	Examples	Effective medication
Nociceptive: somatic	Damage to tissue, soft tissue, or bone; inflammation; trauma	Well localized	Aching, sharp	Pain of arthritis, cancer	Aspirin, NSAIDs, COX-2 inhibitors, opiates
Nociceptive: visceral	Injury or damage to visceral structures, organs	Referred pain, fairly well localized	Aching, sharp	Pain of angina, kidney stones, appendicitis	Opiates, other analgesics
Neuropathic	Damage to nerve tissue, either peripheral or CNS	Nerve distributions, poorly localized with CNS sources	Paresthetic, numb, burning, pins-and-needles	Postherpetic neuralgia, trigeminal neuralgia	Antidepressants, anticonvulsants
Psychogenic	No clear underlying cause; psycho-logical distress	Poorly localized	Vague, sweeping	Somatization disorder	Psychotropic medications, psychotherapy

Note.   CNS = central nervous system; COX-2 = cyclooxygenase-2; NSAID = nonsteroidal anti-inflammatory drug.
Source.   Reprinted from Leo RJ, Singh A: "Pain Management in the Elderly: Use of Psychopharmacologic Agents." *Annals of Long-Term Care: Clinical Care and Aging* 10:37–45, 2002. Used with permission.

Table 2–7.   Common problems encountered by patients with chronic pain

Medical	Problems with access to appropriate care Difficulties in establishing a working relationship with practitioner skilled in pain management
Psychological	Comorbid mood disturbances
Physical	The pain itself Deconditioning resulting from inactivity Medical complications from use of multiple medications
Vocational	Job loss Restrictions from usual types of job activities
Financial	Financial problems arising from job loss, loss of medical coverage, or the cost of medical care
Legal	Litigation related to injuries, workers' compensation, or disability issues
Family	Pain's interference with customary role of the patient, causing others within the family to adopt new roles Limited reserves of energy and time left for other family members' needs (e.g., children's needs, their activities, their schoolwork, etc.) because so much is taken up with pain and the pain patient
Sociocultural	Pain's interference with patient's ability to engage in customary activities and maintain social ties, resulting in significant losses in the patient's social support network

Table 2–8 for a comparison of the two categories). In this subset, patients have a notable preoccupation with pain. For these persons, life revolves around the pain. Activities are forestalled, and work is not pursued. The patients may be thrust into positions of marked dependency on others. Several, perhaps all, aspects of their lives are made contingent on pain experiences or are put off because the patients fear their pain might get worse (Sternbach 1974). For such persons, being a patient is a primary psychosocial state. Life experiences become centered on doctors' visits. If these visits are unsatisfying, patients may develop a history of "doctor shopping." They may seek invasive and diagnostic procedures to confirm the existence of the pain or alleviate their distress. Such patients may display increasing preoccupation with medication use and, possibly, abuse. Numerous psychological factors beset the patient with complex pain, many of which can exacerbate and maintain pain (Weisberg and Clavel 1999).

Table 2–8.   Simple versus complex chronic pain

Simple pain	Complex pain
Pain is clearly defined.	Multiple pain complaints are present.
Patient is easily enlisted into treatment.	Difficulty can be encountered enlisting patient into treatment.
Patient's support systems are stable.	Patient has unstable social systems.
Comorbid psychological factors are easily defined.	Severe complicating psychological factors can be present.
Patient's pain shows some response to medications and treatment.	Patient's pain shows poor response to medications and treatment.
Patient may require short-term psychotherapy or psychological interventions.	Patient may require multidisciplinary treatment approaches, including psychiatric treatment.
Litigation is not central to the patient's presentation.	Litigation is apt to be central to the patient's presentation.

Patients with simple chronic pain may do well with a single pain specialist, with referral as needed to services provided by practitioners in other specialties (e.g., psychiatrists, therapists). Patients with complex pain, on the other hand, can overwhelm a single practitioner. Clearly, such patients need a multidisciplinary approach to their pain, involving the coordinated joint efforts of practitioners in medical, surgical, physical, neurologic, or psychiatric services.

Multiaxial Pain Classification

The International Association for the Study of Pain (1986) has advocated a multiaxial classification of chronic pain, comparable to that used in psychiatric diagnosis. The intention behind the classification system is to standardize diagnosis and facilitate research endeavors in pain treatment. Axis I refers to the body region that is the source of pain (e.g., lower back); Axis II refers to the systemic source whose abnormal functioning produces pain (e.g., neurologic system); Axis III characterizes the pattern of the pain and its temporal characteristics (e.g., 6 months of continuous pain that radiates to the lower extremity); Axis IV refers to the patient's rating of pain intensity and pain duration (e.g., severe); and Axis V refers to the etiology (e.g., intervertebral disk rupture). This classification approach may be useful if it is systematized and employed uniformly. However, the multiaxial system has not yet been required by insurers or universally accepted in clinical circles.

Key Points

- Consistent with a biopsychosocial perspective, pain is multidimensional, with biological (nociceptive and sensory), psychological (cognitive appraisal and suffering), and social (overt behaviors and communicated distress) components.
- The neurophysiologic substrates of the pain experience can be broken down into those elements of pain transmission emanating from peripheral, spinal, and supraspinal processes.
- The mechanisms involved in pain processing within the central nervous system are complex, influenced by the dynamic interaction of neurotransmitters, their receptors, and pain-augmenting and pain-inhibiting neural circuits.
- Awareness of the diverse array of neurophysiologic processes underlying the experience of pain can form the basis for appreciating various modes of intervention for pain treatment. Overlap between neurophysiologic processes underlying pain and related conditions (e.g., depression) may account for the high rates of comorbidity between them.
- Differences between acute and chronic pain have largely been based on the duration of pain. It may be more pertinent to distinguish patients with pain by the extent to which their lives are adversely affected by their symptoms. Thus, in the case of patients with complex pain, one's life becomes centered on pain and disability; being a patient becomes a primary psychosocial state. Multidisciplinary treatment approaches become essential not only to address symptom relief but also to mitigate related mood disturbances, improve adaptive functioning, and reduce the life dissatisfaction that accompanies such complex pain states.

References

Besson JM, Chaouch A: Peripheral and spinal mechanisms of nociception. Physiol Rev 67:67–186, 1987

Byers MR, Bonica JJ: Peripheral pain mechanisms and nociceptor plasticity, in Bonica's Management of Pain, 3rd Edition. Edited by Loeser JD, Butler SH, Chapman CR, et al. Philadelphia, PA, Lippincott Williams & Wilkins, 2001, pp 26–72

Chudler EH, Bonica JJ: Supraspinal mechanisms of pain and nociception, in Bonica's Management of Pain, 3rd Edition. Edited by Loeser JD, Butler SH, Chapman CR, et al. Philadelphia, PA, Lippincott Williams & Wilkins, 2001, pp 153–179

Crue BL: Neurophysiology and taxonomy of pain, in Management of Patients With Chronic Pain. Edited by Brena SF, Chapman SL. New York, Spectrum, 1983, pp 21–31

Dennis SG, Melzack R: Pain-signaling systems in the dorsal and ventral spinal cord. Pain 4:97–132, 1977

Dubner R, Bennett GJ: Spinal and trigeminal mechanisms of nociception. Annu Rev Neurosci 6:381–418, 1983

Giesler GJ, Katter JT, Dado RJ: Direct spinal pathways to the limbic system for nociceptive information. Trends Neurosci 17:244–250, 1994

International Association for the Study of Pain, Subcommittee on Taxonomy: Classification of chronic pain: descriptions of chronic pain syndromes and definitions of pain terms. Pain Suppl 3:S1–S226, 1986

Leo RJ, Singh A: Pain management in the elderly: use of psychopharmacologic agents. Annals of Long-Term Care: Clinical Care and Aging 10:37–45, 2002

Levine JD, Fields HL, Basbaum AI: Peptides and the primary afferent nociceptor. J Neurosci 13:2273–2286, 1993

Loeser JD: Concepts of pain, in Chronic Low Back Pain. Edited by Stanton-Hicks M, Boas R. New York, Raven, 1982, pp 145–148

McMahon SB: Mechanisms of sympathetic pain. Br Med Bull 47:584–600, 1991

Melzack R, Wall PD: Pain mechanisms: a new theory. Science 150:971–979, 1965

Pomeranz B, Wall PD, Weber WV: Cord cells responding to fine myelinated afferents from viscera, muscle, and skin. J Physiol 199:511–532, 1968

Portenoy RK: Mechanisms of clinical pain: observations and speculations. Neurol Clin 7:205–230, 1989

Rome H, Rome J: Limbically augmented pain syndrome (LAPS): kindling, corticolimbic sensitization, and the convergence of affective and sensory symptoms in chronic pain disorders. Pain Med 1:7–23, 2000

Sewell RDE, Lee RL: Opiate receptors, endorphins and drug therapy. Postgrad Med J 56:25–30, 1980

Snyder SH: Brain peptides as neurotransmitters. Science 209:976–983, 1980

Sternbach RA: Pain Patients: Traits and Treatment. New York, Academic Press, 1974

Terenius L: Families of opioid peptides and classes of opioid receptors, in Advances in Pain Research and Therapy, Vol 9. Edited by Fields HL, Dubner R, Cervero F. New York, Raven, 1985, pp 463–477

Terman GW, Bonica JJ: Spinal mechanisms and their modulation, in Bonica's Management of Pain, 3rd Edition. Edited by Loeser JD, Butler SH, Chapman CR, et al. Philadelphia, PA, Lippincott Williams & Wilkins, 2001, pp 73–152

Wall PD: The role of substantia gelatinosa as a gate control. Res Publ Assoc Res Nerv Ment Dis 58:205–231, 1980

Weisberg MB, Clavel AL Jr: Why is chronic pain so difficult to treat? Psychological considerations from simple to complex care. Postgrad Med 106:141–142, 145–148, 157–160, 163–164, 1999

Zimmerman M: Peripheral and central nervous mechanisms of nociception, pain and pain therapy: facts and hypotheses, in Advances in Pain Research and Therapy. Edited by Bonica JJ, Liebeskind JC, Albe-Fessard DG. New York, Raven, 1979, pp 3–32

3

Evaluation of the Pain Patient

Comprehensive assessment of the pain patient involves judicious use of history, physical examination, pain assessments, diagnostic testing, and psychological testing. In this chapter I focus on the elements of comprehensive history gathering. Given that pain is a subjective experience, a number of measurement indices have been employed as part of the assessment that allow for grading the quantity, extent, or severity of the pain. The elements of the history are the focus of the first portion of this chapter, and pain assessments are discussed in the second portion.

The neural processing of pain is quite complex, involving more than just sensory processes. In fact, pain processing involves neurologic substrates common to emotion and cognition (i.e., limbic and cortical systems). The experience of pain and the appreciation of, and reactions to, pain information involve cognitive and emotional factors. The behaviors displayed by the pain patient can likewise have an impact on social and adaptive functioning. It follows, then, that pain assessment can be quite complex, involving somatic and psychological factors (cognitive, emotional, and motivational), as well as adaptive and social functioning (Figure 3–1).

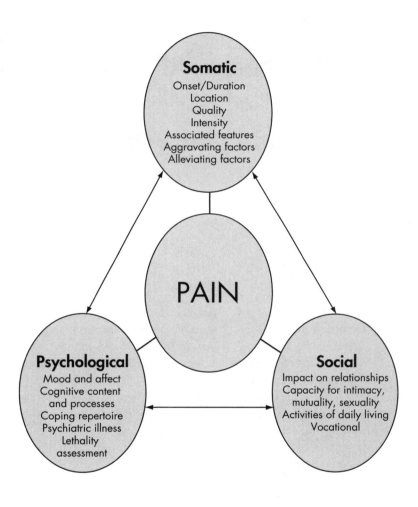

Figure 3–1.   Components of the pain history.

Conducting an Interview

During the course of verbal evaluation, the patient should be encouraged to speak freely. Open-ended lines of inquiry should be employed to prompt the patient to elaborate (e.g., "Tell me more about the pain" or "How has the pain affected your lifestyle?"). Very specific lines of inquiry (e.g., "Is the pain aggravated by movement?") often restrict the free elaboration of the patient, can prematurely limit the patient's willingness to provide information, and can confine the patient's reporting of history to the examiner's persuasion and biases. Open-ended lines of inquiry communicate that the patient is listened to, whereas a litany of questions can suggest that the patient's impressions and experiences of pain are of less importance.

Occasional paraphrased recapitulation of the patient's report allows the interviewer to clarify what was conveyed. If aspects of the history are missing, the practitioner can quickly insert clarifying inquiries (e.g., "Let me see if I got this right. You indicated that you have been experiencing dull, aching pain in your lower back. It seems to radiate down your right leg, and it makes you feel unsteady when you walk. Is that right?"). If the paraphrasing is confirmed, the practitioner might consider redirecting and clarifying questions (e.g., "I am still unclear about something. What seems to bring on the pain?"). With patients who have difficulty articulating characteristics of the pain, encouraging the use of metaphor could facilitate capturing the features of the pain experience (Fishman and Loscalzo 1987).

Patients appear for psychiatric evaluation with varying agendas. For example, a patient might seek out psychiatric assessment at the recommendation of a clinician who is concerned about the patient's adherence to treatment or about psychological issues that might be contributing to or exacerbating pain. On the other hand, the patient might have an agenda that is quite different from the clinician's agenda (e.g., the impact of pain on relationships, employment, and quality of life). The open-ended line of inquiry allows for exposure and examination of the more covert aspects of the patient's reasons for seeking evaluation or treatment. Ascertaining the patient's agenda can be helpful in guiding the interview and arriving at a reasonable treatment plan that reflects the patient's needs. An example: A patient sought help on the recommendation of her physician, who presumed that depression was complicating her chronic back pain. During the evaluation, it became apparent that she had concerns about marital issues arising from role modifications within the home as a result of her pain (e.g., "My husband doesn't understand my pain"). It seemed that more direct attention to facilitating effective patterns of communication, problem solving, and coping within the marriage would be required in order to mitigate both the depression and the back pain.

Obtaining the Pain History

Somatic Component

Essential to the diagnosis of pain disorders is information about the somatic components of the pain: its duration, course, intensity, and precipitating and mitigating factors. The more detailed this history, the more likely it is that the psychiatrist will arrive at an understanding of the pain features amenable to treatment. In addition, clarity of these features allows the clinician to determine whether the interventions and treatments used are effective, because one should be able to detect changes and improvements in some or all of these parameters. Table 3–1 summarizes the somatic components to be obtained in the pain history (Morgan and Engel 1969).

Table 3–1.   Obtaining a pain history

Onset	When did the pain begin?
Location	Where is the pain located? Does it radiate? If so, where? What factors influence the radiation?
Quality	What is the pain like?
Quantity	How intense is the pain?
Duration and chronology	How long has the pain been going on? What has the course of your pain been like? Is it getting better? Worse?
Setting	Under what circumstances does the pain occur?
Aggravating and alleviating factors	What factors aggravate the pain? What brings about relief or attenuation of pain?
Associated features	What other symptoms are associated with the pain? How does it affect your sleep? Your appetite? Your energy level?

Source.   Adapted from Morgan ML, Engel GL: *The Clinical Approach to the Patient.* Philadelphia, PA, WB Saunders, 1969.

Table 3–2. Psychiatric disorders accompanying acute and chronic pain

Anxiety disorders
Delirium
Depression
Sexual dysfunction
Sleep disorders
Somatoform disorders
    Conversion disorder
    Hypochondriasis
    Pain disorder
    Somatization disorder
Substance abuse or dependence

Chronic disorders of any sort, by virtue of their occurrence over time, will produce changes in a person's emotional and psychological state, influence adaptive functioning, and affect social roles and relationships. Thus, evaluation of such patients naturally prompts inquiry into the factors that predispose, activate, and perpetuate the pain and disability. These factors may possibly involve psychosocial stressors. Examination of the factors that render treatment ineffective is also warranted. Once all of these factors are evaluated and addressed, appropriate treatment, rehabilitation, and reclamation of the patient will be possible (Aronoff et al. 2000). Having established the history of pain complaints, the physician can direct attention to the psychological and social correlates of the pain.

Psychological Component

Certainly, any focus on somatic concerns should prompt the psychiatrist to consider psychiatric comorbidities in which pain or other related somatic concerns might be a feature or focus (Fishbain 1999a). Careful inquiry will need to be made into common psychiatric comorbidities associated with pain (Table 3–2).

The psychiatrist should inquire into the relationship of emotional and psychological states to subjective pain complaints and exacerbations. Inquiry should be conducted in a manner that does not trigger defensiveness on the part of the patient. Often, patients have become accustomed to being rejected by physicians who use traditional medical approaches and have felt as though their pain complaints have been dismissed as being all in their head. Consequently, patients with chronic pain can be exquisitely sensitive to inquiry that suggests even the most remote aspects of psychological and emotional dysfunction. They may well fear that attention could be directed away from the physical aspects of treatment. Nonetheless, they could respond favorably to the comprehensiveness of an assessment—including the possible emotional and psychological effects of chronic pain—and the prospect that treatment directed at the psychological factors accompanying pain might also have pain-mitigating effects.

The essential components of the psychological variables related to pain are summarized in Figure 3–1. These items are interrelated, so there is considerable overlap in a person's moods, cognitive appraisals, and coping strategies. Thus, flexibility is required in assessment of each of these components.

Mood and Affect

Careful examination of mood states can begin with inquiry into the patient's pervasive mood over recent weeks and whether this represents a change from his or her baseline mood. Concerned primarily about illness, disability, functioning, and treatment, the patient may well dismiss his or her own mood or affective states as being natural reactions to the pain state. Consequently, inquiry might be directed at how other people in the patient's life have commented on the patient's recent mood and whether they have construed the recent mood as a distinct change from the patient's usual mood.

Inquiry into mood and affective states is likely to reveal the emotional factors related to the pain experiences among patients with chronic pain. Among inpatients with chronic pain, pain ratings were linearly correlated with anger, fear (or anxiety), and depression. On the other hand, the presence of joy, interest, and surprise were predictive of lower pain states. Other emotional states (e.g., shame, disgust, contempt) were only weakly correlated with pain complaints (Fernandez and Milburn 1994).

It might be possible to determine in the interview that certain affective states are temporally related to pain levels. Discrete, situational emotions are important determinants of pain ratings (Gaskin et al. 1992). Thus, for example, it could become apparent that certain emotional states precede pain, whereas other emotional states arise after the experience of pain. Exacerbations of pain could possibly predispose a person to certain affective states (e.g., dysphoria, anxiety, anger) (Huyser and Parker 1999). On the other hand, the presence of affective states (e.g., anger) could possibly result in exacerbations of pain. Thus, dysphoria can arise as a reaction to the pain experience, as a result of the lack of satisfactory treatment, in response to the sequelae of pain, or as an independent disorder (i.e., depression) warranting treatment. It might be helpful to discern whether such relationships exist, because these relationships can have implications for possible treatment interventions.

Anger can be an important component of the experience of the patient with chronic pain (Wade et al. 1990). The presence of anger in and of itself is not a problem. Rather, problems arise when there is a conflict around the expression of anger, there is difficulty around the expression of anger, or there are high levels of hostility. In these circumstances, there is likely to be activation of the autonomic nervous system and endocrine systems (e.g., increased cortisol levels) and other physiologic effects of anger (Fernandez and Turk 1995). Patients incapable of diffusing anger or channeling it into appropriate avenues are prone to resentment, suspicion, mistrust, and heightened levels of arousal. Likewise, inability to modulate unpleasant emotional states is likely to heighten levels of pain (Kinder and Curtiss 1988).

Anxiety disorders are accompanied by an increased incidence of somatic symptoms and pain complaints (Beidel et al. 1991). Anxiety can lower pain thresholds and predispose one to heightened somatic concerns (Barsky et al. 1988).

More important than the mere presence of a particular affective state are the ways in which unpleasant emotional states are managed. Thus, inquiry into coping strategies would be warranted (see also section "Coping Strategies" later in this chapter). Naturally, the repertoire of strategies one employs to comfort oneself and the effectiveness of those strategies would be of interest.

Cognitive Patterns

The psychiatrist needs to examine the patient's cognitions about pain—that is, the beliefs held by the patient about the meaning of the pain, expectations about future pain, and interpretation of the impact the pain has on his or her life, functioning, and relationships. Cognitive appraisal of pain depends on the individual's perspective on the consequences of pain on his or her well-being, the importance he or she assigns to the pain, and his or her view of the measures available to cope with the pain and its ramifications.

Questions arise as to the role the pain plays in the patient's life. This aspect of inquiry might naturally follow from discussions of the medical conditions underlying the pain. The topic can be introduced by asking patients what they were told about the cause of the pain and what their reactions were to these explanations. For example, for some patients the explanations offered by clinicians are reassuring; for others, they are met with incredulity. This line of inquiry can reveal the sorts of preoccupations and concerns about the pain that might not have been overtly expressed to other clinicians. For example, in patients with cancer, this line of inquiry might unveil thoughts the patients have about fears that the cancer is spreading or that it now renders them "terminal." It also can reveal misconceptions about the pain or distortions of what has been disclosed to them and, therefore, a need for clarification and education. When there is no clear etiology for the pain, the interviewer can gain insight into the patient's disease conviction. *Disease conviction* refers to the extent to which patients maintain that they are ill, how much they are bothered by symptoms, and the extent to which they would accept the reassurances of the physician. Disease conviction is notably present among depressed patients with somatic concerns (Pilowsky 1975).

Attention needs to be directed to listening for the distorted cognitive patterns and styles that can be manifested by the patient with pain (Table 3–3). These patterns and styles may be influenced by one's prevailing emotional state. On the other hand, such cognitive patterns can influence one's emotional state. Thus, the relationships are likely to be reciprocal. Such cognitive styles are likely to reduce self-efficacy, hamper development of effective coping, drain one's support systems, accentuate unpleasant emotional states (e.g., anger, anxiety, depression), and exacerbate pain. The presence of such patterns, therefore, could signal the need for psychotherapeutic interventions.

In a recent interview, a distressed patient reported, "The pain—it's always there. It ruins my entire life. There is absolutely nothing that gives me relief." The patterns reflected in these statements signal the presence of catastrophizing ("It ruins my entire life"), overgeneralizing ("It's always there"), and helplessness ("Absolutely nothing that gives me relief"). Recognition of these features might prompt further inquiry into similar beliefs about other aspects of the patient's life. Using this line of inquiry, the evaluator can determine how pervasive these patterns of beliefs are, how rigidly they are maintained, and how malleable the person is in terms of alternative ways of looking at his or her condition.

Table 3–3.   Problematic cognitive patterns in pain

Catastrophizing	Tendency to view and expect the worst (e.g., "I am doomed to have pain and misery forever!")
Helplessness	Belief that nothing that one does matters, that there is no benefit despite one's best efforts (e.g., "My doctor says that I should exercise to improve my osteoarthritis. I know it won't help!")
Help-rejecting	Rejection of the efforts of well-meaning others as a means of expressing anger, securing ongoing support or attention, or even manipulating others (e.g., "I had problems with the last four medicines you gave me.")
Labeling	Ascribing a behavior of a person to a characteristic or nature of the person; the patient who is disappointed about the ineffectiveness of a medication might need to discount the qualifications of the clinician (e.g., "The medication the doctor gave me didn't help. What a quack!")
Magnification	Exaggeration of the significance of a negative event (e.g., "My pain got worse at work yesterday. I had to leave an hour early. I might as well come to grips with the fact that I am totally disabled!")
Overgeneralization	Expanding one adverse event or setback to many or all aspects of one's life (e.g., "If this medication doesn't help me, nothing will!")
Personalization	Interpretation that an event or situation is indicative of something about oneself (e.g., "Because of the pain, I am a worthless failure!")
Selective abstraction	Propensity to attend selectively to negative aspects of one's life while ignoring satisfying and rewarding aspects (e.g., "Everything that happens in my life is bad!")

Coping Strategies

Identification of problematic emotions and cognitive patterns should signal a need for inquiry into the coping strategies used by the individual to self-soothe, self-comfort, reduce distress, and modulate unpleasant states. Inquiry should again be open-ended (e.g., "When you get to feeling [or thinking] this way, how do you cope?"). Attentive listening to active and passive strategies is required. Some patients have a propensity to retreat and withdraw from other people (thus affecting social functioning). Other patients might have a need to enlist and secure the support of others (an approach that can be adaptive or maladaptive). Still other patients have a tendency to engage in passive coping strategies (e.g., hoping for relief, praying, sleeping). For still others, there might be a tendency to distract themselves with other activities, engage in self-statements that can produce relief, and so forth (Rosenstiel and Keefe 1983).

Some patients are apt to focus on somatic complaints and pain, as opposed to dealing with the distress and emotional responses incurred by having a painful condition. In addition, somatic amplification might be invoked when emotionally laden distress is difficult for patients to tolerate or to address directly. Thus, some patients tend instead to focus on, embellish, or magnify somatic complaints and concerns so as to enlist the support of others and to communicate to others their level of distress. Others might cope with unpleasant emotions and cognitive patterns by self-medicating with analgesics or even by abusing substances.

Coping strategies that involve the support of other people may be healthy or they may be overdemanding and exasperating to members of the patient's social support network. Patients' cognitive processes can serve to put up barriers to addressing and dealing with problem areas in their lives. Statements such as "This pain will be the ruin of me! It will never get better, no matter what they tell me to do!" might actually serve to foster passivity and buffer the patient from taking any responsibility in the rehabilitation process.

It is critical to assess lethality. Patients with chronic pain and unremitting or terminal illnesses are particularly prone to despair. The risk of suicide is increased among persons with medical illnesses in which there is distress over disfigurement (Work Group on Suicidal Behaviors 2003), pain (Chochinov et al. 1995; Fishbain 1999b; Fishbain et al. 1991), comorbid mood disorders (Work Group on Suicidal Behaviors 2003), substance abuse (Borges et al. 2000), severe functional impairments (Waern et al. 2002), or increased perceived levels of disability. It is imperative to carefully inquire into thoughts of despair, hopelessness, suicidal ideas and suicide intent, and whether plans are present. In ascertaining the severity of these issues, it is important to determine the following: Is there a history of prior suicide attempt? If so, did the attempt occur within recent months? Is there a family history of suicide? What support systems are in place to ensure the patient's safety? Does the patient make use of those available supports?

Social and Adaptational Component

The patient's social history can be especially important in understanding the profound impact of pain (see Figure 3–1). Another important feature to consider is the patient's adaptive functioning. Inquiry should be focused on what the patient is able to do and what activities are avoided because of the pain. A thorough evaluation of the following factors is indicated: the patient's day-to-day activities and interests, loss of (or decline in) activities due to the pain, the patient's occupation, how work is affected, how the patient is supported (if not by work), concerns over the accessibility and cost of medical care, whether litigation related to the cause of pain is pending, and whether applications for disability are under review. Inquiry into the patient's general life satisfaction is critical (e.g., how free time is spent, pursuit of interests, how the patient comforts himself or herself, how the patient manages pleasant and unpleasant emotions). The interviewer needs to listen for elements that suggest the patient assumes an invalid role in all or most aspects of his or her life and assess the function that role serves for the patient.

Especially pertinent is the identification of significant persons in the patient's life and how the pain has influenced relationships with those persons. For example, pain patients and their significant others can experience loss in intimacy and sexual dissatisfaction because of the impact of pain on sexual functioning.

Inquiry into how pain is communicated to others, the expected responses, the responses generated and from whom, and how the patient perceives those responses is germane. Inquiry should be directed to how the patient's pain influences the behaviors of others. To avoid defensiveness on the part of the patient, the examiner should avoid implying that such influence on others is intentional or manipulative. However, the interviewer should recognize the possibility that such influences may be unconsciously driven. Given that interpersonal relationships are bidirectional, it is equally important to ascertain the extent to which the patient's adaptation in the context of pain may be shaped or reinforced by the responses of others in his or her life (Turk and Okifuji 2002).

Careful histories of alcohol and drug use are imperative. Abused agents can include medications prescribed for the patient's use (e.g., opiate analgesics), and patients may become defensive if they fear that analgesics provided to them—even if not fully effective in eradicating pain—might be withdrawn or withheld. Patients might require assurance that this line of inquiry is part of a comprehensive approach. This inquiry is also important in determining what types of medical and pharmacologic approaches best suit the patients' needs.

Longitudinal Approach

A historical perspective on the pain history can be quite helpful in understanding the evolution of the present pain experience. Thus, it can be useful to evaluate the patient's early pain complaints, history of medical interventions, and response to treatment. There can be indications of the quality of previous doctor–patient interactions; how proactive or passive a role the patient took; and the patient's history of adherence to medical treatment, including physical or occupational therapy, medications, diet, exercise, and other components. Earlier history can constitute a backdrop against which the current pain experiences can be evaluated. Previous experiences can influence the patient's expectations of current treatment, his or her current doctor–patient relationships, and the patient's participation and follow-through with treatment.

Other longitudinal aspects include developmental life experiences. The presence of early childhood illnesses (e.g., diabetes) can have a profound impact on family interactions and the shaping of early relationships. These experiences can shape current relationships as well. Family history of medical illnesses, particularly those involving pain, and how these were experienced by the family—and by the patient in particular—can reveal patterns of pain behaviors with which the patient grew up and that influence current experiences (Fishman and Loscalzo 1987). These patterns may have an impact on how the patient currently manages his or her pain. Degree of impairment and disability arising from painful medical or surgical conditions can also have been "learned" by the patient in such early experiences. Responses of family members to treatment endeavors might have shaped the patient's expectations and beliefs about the utility and effectiveness of pain interventions, whether or not those early experiences bore directly on the type of pain (or the source of pain) the patient experiences in his or her own current medical condition.

Other developmental factors may have an impact on a person's current social and adaptive functioning. For example, a history of sexual abuse is present in a number of patients with chronic pelvic pain, abdominal pain, and even disorders such as fibromyalgia (Gross et al. 1980). Accessing this information can relay significant history about the dynamics within the home, how crises were managed, what support systems were available to the patient while growing up, and whether the patient has a support system in place to actually support, nurture, and protect him or her. This inquiry should be conducted in a sensitive and respectful manner. Patients may well be reluctant to confide such information, fearing that it could reflect adversely on them. They may feel a need or a desire to protect family members despite the abuse itself or the family's failure to intervene on their behalf even in the face of evidence or suggestion of abuse. Patients may need to be informed that such experiences can influence how they approach their world, can affect the patients' expectations regarding the reliability and goodwill of treating sources (authority figures), and have been related to certain chronic pain disorders.

Evaluation of Treatment Suitability

At times, psychiatric evaluation is requested to assess the factors that contribute barriers to effective pain treatment. Evaluation can determine whether psychopharmacologic treatment, psychotherapeutic modalities, or both should be employed. Sometimes psychiatric evaluation is requested when psychological factors are mediating the pain experience or when psychiatric disorders more completely explain the origin of the pain. Psychiatric evaluation can be conducted to assess the patient's suitability for other interventions (e.g., surgery). Table 3–4 lists the factors that predict a poor surgical outcome for pain disorders. Once such factors are addressed in psychiatric treatment, however, a patient could possibly be considered for surgical interventions (see also section "Role of the Psychiatrist in Pain Management Related to Interventions" in Chapter 7, "Special Techniques in Pain Management," of this book).

Pain Assessment Instruments

Pain assessment tests and scales are useful adjuncts to the evaluation of the pain patient. These instruments allow the examiner to ascertain the severity and intensity of the pain experience. A number of scales are available, and the selection of the assessment instrument to be used is determined in part by the characteristics of the pain and the elements gleaned from the interview (see Table 3–5 for a list of psychometric scales used in assessing chronic pain). In acute pain states, certain types of assessments are desirable that are of limited utility in assessing chronic pain states (see Table 3–6 for a summary of the

Table 3–4.   Factors that suggest poor surgical outcome for pain disorders

Emotional factors
  Anger
  Anxiety
  Depression
Cognitive factors
  Catastrophizing
  Perception of loss of control
Vocational factors
  Financial settlement or pending litigation
  Job dissatisfaction
  Workers' compensation
Social factors
  Marital dissatisfaction
Historical factors
  History of physical abuse
  History of sexual abuse
  Prior psychological treatment
  Substance abuse or dependence

instruments used in acute vs. chronic pain). On the other hand, multidimensional pain assessments and complex behavioral assessments can be invoked when complex interactions between pain states and psychosocial factors are implicated in mediating pain.

   Patients with acute pain (e.g., postoperative pain) are preoccupied with the situational characteristics of the pain. The pain is expected to be time limited. Conversely, for those with chronic pain, their day-to-day, interpersonal, academic, and vocational functioning are overshadowed by the pain experience. Therefore, assessments used in acute pain settings will be fundamentally different from those used in chronic pain. Measures for acute pain, summarized in Table 3–6, focus on the experience and intensity of pain and assess responsiveness to treatment interventions. Chronic pain assessments focus on broader aspects of patients' pain experiences, functioning, and psychological adaptation.

   The pain assessments described in the following subsections serve a number of functions, including assessment of pain intensity, quality, and duration. In addition, such scales can assist the physician in making treatment selections and assessing the efficacy of treatment.

Table 3–5. Psychometric scales used in assessing chronic pain

Coping Strategies Questionnaire	Assesses the coping strategies in patient's repertoire to deal with chronic pain. May predict the level of activity, physical impairment, and psychological functioning associated with pain.
Fear-Avoidance Beliefs Questionnaire	Assesses beliefs characterized by danger, threat, or harm associated with pain. The degree to which patients assign threat to activities can limit their participation in, and lead to avoidance of, activities related to work.
McGill Pain Questionnaire	Assesses the features of pain severity and intensity. Allows patients to qualify pain in emotional, cognitive-evaluative, and sensory terms.
Minnesota Multiphasic Personality Inventory	Provides personality profile and pathologic assessment of patient with chronic pain.
Pain Interference Indices	Assess the impact of chronic pain states on various aspects of a person's activity, functioning, and role responsibilities.
Multidimensional Pain Inventory	Assesses patient's appraisal of pain, its impact on his or her functioning, and the patient's perceived responses of others to his or her pain.

Single-Dimension Scales

The most commonly used pain scales involve single-dimension ratings of pain intensity. Such scales are appealing because of their ease of administration and interpretation. Patients also find them easy to complete (e.g., requiring little in the way of time commitment or concentration). However, single-dimension scales have been criticized for oversimplifying pain ratings and for ignoring factors that contribute to or exacerbate the pain experience (e.g., emotional and cognitive factors).

Verbal Descriptor Scale

A verbal descriptor scale (VDS) requires that a patient rate the pain experienced according to one of five to seven verbal descriptors. Only limited types of responses are permitted. Such scales can be used in clinical and experimental settings. Of course, use of a VDS assumes that the patient has intact verbal skills (i.e., reading and comprehension). Thus, these measures may not be useful for patients who have significant language barriers or cognitive impairments or for

Table 3–6.   Pain assessment instruments for acute and chronic pain

Acute pain	Recurrent/chronic pain
Visual analog scale or numeric rating scale	Visual analog scale, McGill Pain Questionnaire
Medication use	Medication use
Observer rating	Observer rating
	Pain diary
	Multidimensional Pain Inventory
	Psychological measures

young children. The scoring of a VDS correlates with pain ratings of other scales (e.g., a visual analog scale [VAS]). The VDS, included in Figure 3–2, ignores the emotional, cognitive, and behavioral components of pain.

Numeric Rating Scale

A numeric rating scale (NRS) is often used to measure pain experience and intensity. Patients are asked to rate their pain on an 11-point scale, from 0 (no pain) to 10 (worst pain). A variation of this scale shows a rating of pain from 0 to 100, with similar anchors (Jensen et al. 1986). These scales are reliable and correlate with other simple assessment measures. Use of an NRS requires that the patient have intact language and cognitive skills. One drawback of NRSs is that the patient's rating of pain (i.e., the number selected) has no intrinsic meaning. Thus, if a patient rates his pain as a 5, this rating cannot be assumed to be one-half that of another patient who rates her pain as a 10. Furthermore, the transition from one rating (e.g., from 5 to 4) might not mean the same, even within the same patient, as a transition at another point in the scale (e.g., from 9 to 8).

Visual Analog Scale

An extension of NRSs, the Visual Analogue Scale consists of a 10-cm line with anchors at 0 and 10 or verbal anchors (see Figure 3–2). The patient is asked to draw an X along the line that best denotes his or her level of pain. The VAS has been used in clinical as well as experimental settings. The denoted pain levels for an individual can be compared over time to quantify levels of pain worsening or improving. These serial comparisons, unlike those employed with repeated use of NRSs, are proportional. However, the use of the VAS for clinical compari-

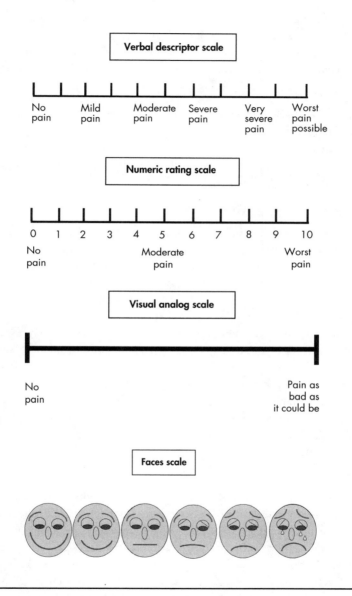

Figure 3–2. Single-dimension pain assessment instruments.

sons has been questioned (Carlsson 1983). A VAS might not be suitable for elderly patients or patients who have difficulty understanding its abstract concept. In such cases, pain can be erroneously denoted, and the faulty values can impede the appropriate characterization of the pain and its treatment.

Faces Scale

With the faces scale, the patient is asked to rate pain intensity according to printed facial expressions conveying varying amounts of distress (see Figure 3–2). This is an easily understood rating instrument and one that has appeal for children. The faces scale allows the examiner to bypass issues related to language barriers (Frank et al. 1982).

Behavioral Measures

Behavioral measures are instruments that assess pain in a manner vastly different from the simple rating scales. Although some professionals in the field have questioned the utility and reliability of observer ratings of pain behavior, these ratings are often used by clinicians and nursing staff. Thus, when someone complains of distress, the clinician often examines the overt behavior of the patient to look for corroborating behaviors that substantiate the allegation of pain. The clinician might look for evidence of distress, facial grimacing, wincing or frowning, guarding of an affected area, limping, splinting, muscle tension, and similar behaviors. The problem with observer ratings is that the results are contingent upon the skill of the observer in detecting pain symptoms. However, observer ratings are also subject to a great deal of bias. For instance, observing a patient with chronic pain who is able to smile or make puns periodically might lead one to dismiss the patient's allegations of pain because of the bias that such behaviors would be entirely inconsistent with pain.

Medication Use

Reviews of the patient's use of medications can be an indicator of the patient's pain experience and severity. It is useful to assess the patient's adherence to treatment, appropriateness of medication use, and excess medication use. Pain patients can be unreliable about medication use and can significantly underestimate the extent of their opioid use (Ready et al. 1982). Thus, the support of collateral informants (e.g., from a spouse or other family member) to provide information about the use of medications can be helpful.

Pain Diary

A pain diary can be as simple or as detailed as the clinician deems necessary (see Figure 3–3 for an example). Categories that might be included in a pain diary include the date and time; the pain rating; the situation; the patient's emotions, behavior, and thoughts; and the response of others to the patient's pain. Pain diaries can be very useful, revealing patterns of pain intensity, exacerbations of pain, and mitigating factors. They can likewise uncover varying psychological states temporally related to episodes of pain or pain relief. This information can be particularly useful when patients are resistant to the idea that psychological states could be related to the pain experience. Also, diaries can be a source of information about the extent to which patients engage in activities (e.g., reclining, pursuing their interests).

Completion of pain diaries can be quite time-consuming for patients. For the diary to be maximally effective, the patient must be committed to maintaining it. Completion of the entire diary for a week in the hour preceding the doctor's appointment limits the utility of the diary, because the entries will be based on the patient's memory and recollections. Instead, the utility of the diary is best derived when the patient maintains the diary reliably and consistently during the periods of study. However, the more complex the diary, the less inclined the patient might be to reliably make entries, because the task can seem overwhelming. In addition, clinicians need to devote some time to review the diary contents to look for trends in the pain ratings and associated temporal features.

Multidimensional Pain Scales

McGill Pain Questionnaire

In the McGill Pain Questionnaire (MPQ; Melzack 1975), a verbal rating scale commonly used to characterize pain, subjects are asked to select verbal descriptors for their pain among sets of categories of descriptors. A long form and short form are available for use. The long form contains 20 sets of categories. The first 10 sets of descriptors refer to the sensory-discriminative aspects of the pain. Sets 11–15 contain items that characterize the affective-emotional components of the pain. Set 16 contains descriptors that correspond to the evaluative components of pain, and the remaining sets (17–20) contain miscellaneous items. The short form of the MPQ (see Table 3–7) contains 15 items.

Date/Time	Pain rating	Situation	Mood/Affect	Activity	Thoughts	Response of others

Figure 3–3. Example of a pain diary format.

Table 3–7. Short form of the McGill Pain Questionnaire

	None	Mild	Moderate	Severe
Throbbing	0)_____	1)_____	2)_____	3)_____
Shooting	0)_____	1)_____	2)_____	3)_____
Stabbing	0)_____	1)_____	2)_____	3)_____
Sharp	0)_____	1)_____	2)_____	3)_____
Cramping	0)_____	1)_____	2)_____	3)_____
Gnawing	0)_____	1)_____	2)_____	3)_____
Hot–burning	0)_____	1)_____	2)_____	3)_____
Aching	0)_____	1)_____	2)_____	3)_____
Heavy	0)_____	1)_____	2)_____	3)_____
Tender	0)_____	1)_____	2)_____	3)_____
Splitting	0)_____	1)_____	2)_____	3)_____
Tiring–exhausting	0)_____	1)_____	2)_____	3)_____
Sickening	0)_____	1)_____	2)_____	3)_____
Fearful	0)_____	1)_____	2)_____	3)_____
Punishing–cruel	0)_____	1)_____	2)_____	3)_____

Source. Reprinted from *Pain,* Volume 30, Melzack R: "The Short-Form McGill Pain Questionnaire," pp. 191–197, 1987. Copyright 1984, with permission from Dr. R. Melzack, McGill University and the International Association for the Study of Pain.

The patient is asked to rank the extent to which each item corresponds to the intensity of his or her pain (Melzack 1987). The short form offers the advantage of being easier to complete, and the scoring correlates with results obtained in the longer form. The MPQ has been translated into a number of different languages for patients for whom language barriers impede the reading or understanding of the English version.

Pain Interference

Any assessment of pain level—or of pain relief resulting from treatment—is less meaningful without a consideration of the patient's perception of the extent to which pain impairs activity and social functioning. Thus, any reductions in pain ratings that suggest an intervention is successful mean little without commensurate changes in the patient's psychological and social well-being and changes in adaptive functions. Examples of such instruments include the Pain Disability Index (Pollard 1984) and the Oswestry Disability Questionnaire (Fairbank et al. 1980). Factors included in such indices include ratings of ability to perform activities of daily living and other customary role responsibilities. These issues can be the basis for modifications in pain treatment and can also be the focus of psychotherapeutic endeavors.

Psychological Assessments

Multidimensional Pain Inventory

The Multidimensional Pain Inventory (MPI) (formerly referred to as the West Haven–Yale Multidimensional Pain Inventory; Kerns et al. 1985) is a 52-item inventory developed for the assessment of a patient's idiosyncratic appraisals of chronic pain. The instrument relies on components of the cognitive-behavioral approach to help understand and conceptualize pain. The instrument is used to examine a person's perceptions, appraisals, and emotions and behaviors associated with pain. Coping strategies used by the individual patient are also assessed, as are the patient's reactions to the responses of others to pain complaints. Not only does the MPI enable the examiner to understand the patient's view of his or her own pain, but it can also serve as a basis for the development of treatment interventions (e.g., to be used in psychotherapy).

Response patterns can reveal patient profiles that might become a focus of clinical attention. A dysfunctional profile reveals high levels of perceived pain, life interference from the pain, low levels of perceived life control, and subjective distress. An interpersonally distressed profile is likewise characterized by high levels of perceived pain and life interference, and patients with this profile perceive themselves as having low levels of social support. Last, an adaptive profile is one in which the patient perceives high levels of self-control, along with low levels of perceived pain and perceived life interference from the pain. The profiles summarized here can have predictive value in terms of treatment approaches and treatment outcomes (Bradley and McKendree-Smith 2001).

Fear-Avoidance Beliefs Questionnaire

The Fear-Avoidance Beliefs Questionnaire (FABQ; Waddell et al. 1993) is a 16-item instrument that assesses the beliefs and fears a patient associates with back pain. Each item is ranked along a 7-point Likert scale that ranges from "strongly agree" to "strongly disagree." The patient's beliefs and fears can have an impact on his or her range and extent of activity. The FABQ assesses fears the patient has about eliciting pain through behaviors required at work and in general activity. The higher the level of fear, the higher the level of the patient's perceived disability.

Coping Strategies Questionnaire

The Coping Strategies Questionnaire (Rosenstiel and Keefe 1983) is useful in assessing active (e.g., diverting one's attention, increasing the level of activity) and passive (e.g., praying, hoping, ignoring pain) coping strategies used by patients dealing with chronic pain. The instrument measures the extent to which maladaptive strategies (e.g., catastrophizing) or more adaptive strategies (e.g., reinterpreting the meaning of the pain and using coping self-statements) are employed. Thus, the scale can illustrate those strategies that are effective and that, therefore, should be maximized when dealing with pain. In addition, those strategies that are ineffective and maladaptive can be the focus of therapeutic interventions to foster modification of those strategies.

Minnesota Multiphasic Personality Inventory

The Minnesota Multiphasic Personality Inventory (MMPI; Hathaway et al. 1989) has been used extensively as an assessment tool for a variety of psychological disturbances. It is also among the most widely used assessment instruments in pain syndromes. The MMPI consists of 566 statements requiring true or false responses. The MMPI comprises 10 standard clinical scales assessing psychopathologic states, 3 validity scales, and 4 additional scales evaluating ego strength and other factors. Consultation with a psychologist trained in the administration and interpretation of the MMPI can be very helpful in the use of this instrument.

The MMPI's strength is its usefulness in identifying psychological factors that warrant clinical attention (e.g., drawing attention to those characteristics that might present barriers to treatment and that ultimately could require psychotherapeutic intervention) (see Table 3–8). The three scales that have the most relevance to patients with pain are Hypochondriasis (Scale 1), Depression (Scale 2), and Hysteria (Scale 3). High scores on Scale 1 suggest that patients, when emotionally distressed, symptomatically channel the distress into somatic complaints. Scale 2 may be an indicator of general distress, but elevated ratings on this scale can suggest a possible depressive disorder. Elevations on Scale 2 may suggest one is unhappy, pessimistic, and self-deprecating. Patients who score high on Scale 3 are characterologically prone to react by developing physical

Table 3–8.   Uses of the Minnesota Multiphasic Personality
Inventory for patients with chronic pain

Can be useful for

    Identifying personality traits/temperament

    Clarifying emotional characteristics

    Clarifying psychological functioning of the patient

    Determining whether psychological factors play a significant role in the pain

Should **not** be used

    For determining "real" versus functional (i.e., "psychogenic") pain

    As a stand-alone prescreening assessment of surgical or other treatment
    interventions

    For predicting response outcomes for surgical or other treatment interventions

symptoms when confronted with stress or uncomfortable emotions. Scales 1 and 3 are often related (Trimboli and Kilgore 1983).

The two most common patterns noted among patients with chronic pain are the *conversion* V and the *neurotic triad* (see Figure 3–4). In the conversion V pattern, elevated ratings on Scales 1 and 3, relative to that on Scale 2, form a valley or V shape when represented on an MMPI graphic profile. Despite use of the term *conversion,* it was never maintained that the pain complaints characterized features of a conversion disorder. Rather, persons with this profile endorse somatic concerns, develop physical complaints in the face of stress, often deny depressive symptoms, and often lack insight into their emotional states (Trimboli and Kilgore 1983). By contrast, those with the neurotic triad pattern (i.e., with elevations on each of the three scales) have somatic preoccupations and neurovegetative symptoms of depression and are often demanding and complaining.

MMPI profiles may change as a patient makes the transition from acute to chronic pain, suggesting commensurate changes in the patient's psychological state over time. The MMPI patterns are modifiable with successful treatment (Naliboff et al. 1988).

Finally, although some empirical work has suggested that the MMPI can be useful in predicting response outcome to treatment interventions (e.g., surgery), its use has not uniformly demonstrated predictive value in this regard (Block et al. 2003). One argument against the interpretation of chronic pain profiles rests with the contention that the items of the MMPI have intrinsic bias—that the Hypochondriasis, Hysteria, and Depression scale items would be endorsed

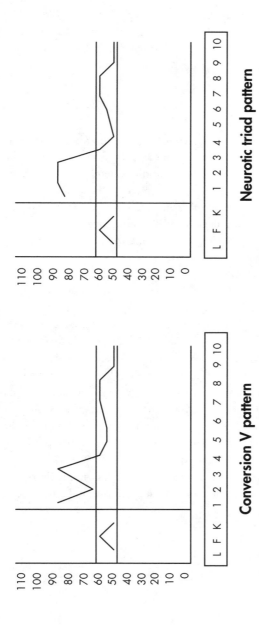

Figure 3–4. Common Minnesota Multiphasic Personality Inventory–2 profiles in chronic pain.

Note. In the first graph, the conversion V pattern is depicted by elevations in scales 1 (Hypochondriasis), 2 (Depression), and 3 (Hysteria), but with depression scores less than those of the other two scales creating a valley. In the second graph, the neurotic triad pattern is depicted by elevations in all three scales.

L, Lie Scale; F, Infrequency Scale; K, Suppressor Scale; 1, Hypochondriasis; 2, Depression; 3, Hysteria; 4, Psychopathic Deviance; 5, Masculinity–Femininity; 6, Paranoia; 7, Psychasthenia; 8, Schizophrenia; 9, Hypomania; 10, Social Introversion.

simply by virtue of the fact that the person is in pain (Smythe 1984). The endorsed items might simply replicate the patient's pain complaints and might not fundamentally characterize a personality prototype of the patient with chronic pain, nor would they necessarily predict treatment response.

Key Points

- Pain assessment needs to be individualized, comprehensive, measurable, and documented sufficiently such that all providers involved in the patient's care have a clear understanding of the patient's pain experiences.
- On a basic level, the clinician needs to characterize the type and intensity of pain. In addition, comprehensive pain assessment requires evaluation of the cognitive, emotional, and social factors influencing the pain experience. Identification of such influences of the pain experience can identify additional areas warranting treatment.
- Psychological factors influencing the pain experience can include disturbances in mood and affect, cognitive appraisals, and coping strategies.
- Social factors influencing the pain experience can include adaptive functioning, the impact of pain on interpersonal relationships, access to medical care, financial and litigation issues, and substance abuse or dependence.
- Standardized instruments allow for quantifiable assessments that, in many cases, are reproducible and reliable. Several single-dimension pain assessment instruments are available that assist with the quantification of pain severity and intensity. Use of multidimensional assessments and psychological instruments can enhance the information gathered from the clinical interview, revealing emotional, cognitive, and subsyndromal psychological factors contributing to the pain experience.
- Together, physical, psychological, and social factors can predispose one to pain, precipitate pain, augment or mitigate pain, and influence one's reactions to pain.

References

Aronoff GM, Tota-Faucette M, Phillips L, et al: Are pain disorder and somatization disorder valid diagnostic entities? Curr Rev Pain 4:309–312, 2000

Barsky AJ, Geringer E, Wool CA: A cognitive-educational treatment for hypochondriasis. Gen Hosp Psychiatry 10:322–327, 1988

Beidel DC, Christ MAG, Long PJ: Somatic complaints in anxious children. J Abnorm Child Psychol 19:659–670, 1991

Block AR, Gatchel RJ, Deardorff WW, et al: The Psychology of Spine Surgery. Washington, DC, American Psychological Association, 2003

Borges G, Walters EE, Kessler RC: Association of substance use, abuse and dependence with subsequent suicidal behavior. Am J Epidemiol 151:781–789, 2000

Bradley LA, McKendree-Smith NL: Assessment of psychological status using interviews and self-report instruments, in Handbook of Pain Assessment, 2nd Edition. Edited by Turk DC, Melzack R. New York, Guilford, 2001, pp 292–319

Carlsson AM: Assessment of chronic pain, I: aspects of the reliability and validity of the visual analogue scale. Pain 16:87–101, 1983

Chochinov HM, Wilson KG, Enns M, et al: Desire for death in the terminally ill. Am J Psychiatry 152:1185–1191, 1995

Fairbank JC, Couper J, Davies JB, et al: The Oswestry low back pain disability questionnaire. Physiotherapy 66:271–273, 1980

Fernandez E, Milburn TW: Sensory and affective predictors of overall pain and emotions associated with affective pain. Clin J Pain 10:3–9, 1994

Fernandez E, Turk DC: The scope and significance of anger in the experience of chronic pain. Pain 61:165–175, 1995

Fishbain DA: Approaches to treatment decisions for psychiatric comorbidity in the management of the chronic pain patient. Med Clin North Am 83:737–760, 1999a

Fishbain DA: The association of chronic pain and suicide. Semin Clin Neuropsychiatry 4:221–227, 1999b

Fishbain DA, Goldberg M, Rosomoff RS, et al: Completed suicide in chronic pain. Clin J Pain 7:29–36, 1991

Fishman B, Loscalzo M: Cognitive-behavioral interventions in management of cancer pain: principles and applications. Med Clin North Am 71:271–287, 1987

Frank AJM, Moll JMH, Hort JF: A comparison of three ways of measuring pain. Rheumatol Rehabil 21:211–217, 1982

Gaskin ME, Greene AF, Robinson ME, et al: Negative affect and the experience of chronic pain. J Psychosom Res 36:707–713, 1992

Gross RJ, Doerr H, Caldirola D, et al: Borderline syndrome and incest in chronic pelvic pain patients. Int J Psychiatry Med 10:79–96, 1980

Hathaway SR, McKinley JC, Butcher JN, et al: Minnesota Multiphasic Personality Inventory–2: Manual for Administration. Minneapolis, University of Minnesota Press, 1989

Huyser BA, Parker JC: Negative affect and pain in arthritis. Rheum Dis Clin North Am 25:105–121, 1999

Jensen MP, Karoly P, Braver S: The measurement of clinical pain intensity: a comparison of six methods. Pain 27:117–126, 1986

Kerns RD, Turk DC, Rudy TE: The West Haven–Yale Multidimensional Pain Inventory (WHYMPI). Pain 23:345–356, 1985

Kinder BN, Curtiss G: Assessment of anxiety, depression and anger in chronic pain patients: conceptual and methodological issues, in Advances in Personality Assessment. Edited by Speilberger CD, Butcher JN. Hillsdale, NJ, Erlbaum, 1988, pp 161–174

Melzack R: The McGill Pain Questionnaire: major properties and scoring methods. Pain 1:277–299, 1975

Melzack R: The Short-Form McGill Pain Questionnaire. Pain 30:191–197, 1987

Morgan ML, Engel GL: The Clinical Approach to the Patient. Philadelphia, PA, WB Saunders, 1969

Naliboff BD, McCreary CP, McArthur DL, et al: MMPI changes following behavioral treatment of chronic low back pain. Pain 35:271–277, 1988

Pilowsky I: Dimensions of abnormal illness behaviour. Aust N Z J Psychiatry 9:141–147, 1975

Pollard CA: Preliminary validity study of the Pain Disability Index. Percept Mot Skills 59:974, 1984

Ready LB, Sarkis E, Turner JA: Self-reported vs. actual use of medications in chronic pain patients. Pain 12:285–294, 1982

Rosenstiel AK, Keefe FJ: The use of coping strategies in chronic low back pain patients: relationship to patient characteristics and current adjustment. Pain 17:33–44, 1983

Smythe HA: Problems with the MMPI. J Rheumatol 11:417–418, 1984

Trimboli FK, Kilgore RB: A psychodynamic approach to MMPI interpretation. J Pers Assess 47:614–626, 1983

Turk DC, Okifuji A: Psychological factors in chronic pain: evolution and revolution. J Consult Clin Psychol 70:678–690, 2002

Waddell G, Newton M, Henderson I, et al: A Fear-Avoidance Beliefs Questionnaire (FABQ) and the role of fear-avoidance beliefs in chronic low back pain and disability. Pain 52:157–168, 1993

Wade JB, Price DD, Hamer RM, et al: An emotional component analysis of chronic pain. Pain 40:303–310, 1990

Waern M, Rubenowitz E, Runeson B, et al: Burden of illness and suicide in elderly people: case-control study. BMJ 324:1355–1357, 2002

Work Group on Suicidal Behaviors: Practice guideline for the assessment and treatment of patients with suicidal behaviors. Am J Psychiatry 160 (11 suppl):1–60, 2003

4

Common Psychiatric Comorbidities and Psychiatric Differential Diagnosis of the Pain Patient

Chronic pain rarely presents alone. Patients with chronic pain tend to have multiple comorbidities that warrant medical attention. The psychiatrist enlisted to care for the patient with chronic pain must consider an extensive psychiatric differential diagnosis. The psychiatric diagnosis can be carefully extracted on the basis of the patient's symptoms, the notable signs during evaluation and interview, the longitudinal course, and supporting evidence provided by laboratory investigations and physical examination. By building on the biopsychosocial approach to pain management outlined in the previous chapter, a thorough psychiatric assessment can enhance understanding of the psychological conditions mediating the pain experience and raise awareness of psychiatric comorbidities that require appropriate treatment.

Pain Disorder

Pain disorder requires that pain be a primary symptom and be severe enough to warrant clinical attention. Marked disability might be alleged, and the patient's life becomes centered on the pain.

Earlier versions of the *Diagnostic and Statistical Manual of Mental Disorders* (DSM) required that clinicians infer whether psychological underpinnings or conflicts precipitated pain complaints. Thus, if it was evident from physical examination and diagnostic evaluation that a physical cause could not fully account for the pain, psychiatric labels were invoked that reflected the psychological origins of the pain—for example, psychogenic pain disorder from DSM-III (American Psychiatric Association 1980) and somatoform pain disorder from DSM-III-R (American Psychiatric Association 1987).

In DSM-IV (American Psychiatric Association 1994) there was a transition in the thinking underlying the diagnosis of pain disorder. The terms *somatoform* and *psychogenic* were dropped. There was no longer a requirement for exclusion of a physical cause for the pain, and the primacy of psychological factors (i.e., conflicts, defenses, and emotional states) underlying and accounting for pain was de-emphasized. DSM-IV-TR (American Psychiatric Association 2000) leaves open the possibility that psychological factors can contribute to the pain experience by precipitating, exacerbating, or maintaining pain, but they do not necessarily have to fully account for the pain. This approach is more consistent with current views of the interrelationships between pain and psychological factors. The DSM-IV-TR diagnostic criteria for pain disorder are presented in Table 4–1.

Pain disorder can be associated with a general medical condition, psychological factors, or both. Pain disorder associated with a general medical condition is recorded solely on Axis III, because psychological factors are thought to have minimal or no involvement in the pain experience. When psychological factors are implicated and are believed to have a significant contributory role in the pain, one of the two other types of pain disorder would be coded on Axis I. However, questions arise as to whether the subtypes represent clinically useful subclassifications. (For example, Aigner and Bach [1999] determined that patients with pain who were categorized into subtypes with psychological versus psychological and general medical features could not be distinguished in terms of pain severity or disability measures.)

Table 4–1. DSM-IV-TR diagnostic criteria for pain disorder

A. Pain in one or more anatomical sites is the predominant focus of the clinical presentation and is of sufficient severity to warrant clinical attention.

B. The pain causes clinically significant distress or impairment in social, occupational, or other important areas of functioning.

C. Psychological factors are judged to have an important role in the onset, severity, exacerbation, or maintenance of the pain.

D. The symptom or deficit is not intentionally produced or feigned (as in factitious disorder or malingering).

E. The pain is not better accounted for by a mood, anxiety, or psychotic disorder and does not meet criteria for dyspareunia.

Code as follows:

> **307.80 Pain Disorder Associated With Psychological Factors:** psychological factors are judged to have the major role in the onset, severity, exacerbation, or maintenance of the pain. (If a general medical condition is present, it does not have a major role in the onset, severity, exacerbation, or maintenance of the pain.) This type of pain disorder is not diagnosed if criteria are also met for somatization disorder.

Specify if:

> **Acute:**   duration of less than 6 months
> **Chronic:**   duration of 6 months or longer

> **307.89 Pain Disorder Associated With Both Psychological Factors and a General Medical Condition:**   both psychological factors and a general medical condition are judged to have important roles in the onset, severity, exacerbation, or maintenance of the pain. The associated general medical condition or anatomical site of the pain (see below) is coded on Axis III.

Specify if:

> **Acute:**   duration of less than 6 months
> **Chronic:**   duration of 6 months or longer

Note: The following is not considered to be a mental disorder and is included here to facilitate differential diagnosis.

Pain Disorder Associated With a General Medical Condition: a general medical condition has a major role in the onset, severity, exacerbation, or maintenance of the pain. (If psychological factors are present, they are not judged to have a major role in the onset, severity, exacerbation, or maintenance of the pain.) The diagnostic code for the pain is selected based on the associated general medical condition if one has been established (see Appendix G) or on the anatomical location of the pain if the underlying general medical condition is not yet clearly established—for example, low back (724.2), sciatic (724.3), pelvic (625.9), headache (784.0), facial (784.0), chest (786.50), joint (719.40), bone (733.90), abdominal (789.0), breast (611.71), renal (788.0), ear (388.70), eye (379.91), throat (784.1), tooth (525.9), and urinary (788.0).

Source.   Reprinted with permission from American Psychiatric Association 2000.

Table 4–2.   Limitations of the DSM-IV-TR nosology of pain disorder

Criteria are not sufficiently operationalized; specifically, there are no guidelines that
allow one to determine
   Whether psychological factors "have an important role" in pain (criterion C).
   When pain is "not better accounted for" by a mood disorder (criterion E).
   Whether, and to what extent, psychological factors are involved in the patient's
   pain.
The nosology of pain disorder is likely to be misunderstood by nonpsychiatric
clinicians.
The characteristics of pain patients can overlap considerably with those of patients
with other somatoform disorders.

Although improved over previous versions, there are several limitations of
the DSM-IV-TR taxonomy (see Table 4–2). In contrast to criteria for many
other psychiatric disorders, the criteria for pain disorder often are perceived as
insufficiently defined, lacking a checklist of symptoms that collectively delineate the syndrome. Thus, for example, there are no guidelines allowing one to
ascertain whether pain is "not better accounted for" by a mood disorder (Sullivan 2000); in fact, it can be quite difficult to make this determination given
the high comorbidity of mood disturbances with pain, as discussed in the section "Depression"). Similarly, an inference is still required on the part of the
clinician to determine whether and to what extent psychological factors are involved in the patient's plight.

By being grouped under the rubric of somatoform disorders, pain disorder
may still connote the implied mind-body dualism of other somatoform disorders (i.e., somatic preoccupation occurring in the absence of, or in excess of,
what would be expected, given objective findings). As a result, the nosology of
pain disorder is likely to be misunderstood by nonpsychiatric clinicians (Mayou
et al. 2003); the potential pejorative implication may be that the patient is dis-
ingenuous, exaggerating, or faking. Ironically, the intent of redefining pain
disorder in DSM-IV-TR was to overcome this archaic dualism.

Pain Disorder Versus Other Somatoform Disorders

Discrepancies arise among diagnosticians when it comes to the psychiatric differential diagnosis accompanying pain. In one review of patients with chronic
pain, somatoform disorders were diagnosed in 16%–53% of the patients (Dwor-

kin and Caligor 1988). In another series, approximately 40% of 283 patients with chronic pain received a diagnosis of conversion disorder (Fishbain et al. 1986). Part of the discrepancy may be due to the diagnostic criteria employed—that is, some diagnoses may have been based on earlier DSM versions in which distinctions among the psychiatric conditions might have been less clear. In addition, sampling bias (i.e., studying patients from very distinct subsets of the population) may have contributed to the diagnostic inconsistencies (Fishbain 1999).

Any pain complaint would not necessarily invoke a diagnosis of pain disorder; rather, it must be considered among a number of other psychiatric disorders in which pain can be a prominent complaint (see Table 4–3). Distinguishing pain disorder from other psychiatric disorders is pertinent to determining appropriate pharmacologic and psychotherapeutic treatment. Nonetheless, the characteristics of pain patients can overlap considerably with those of patients with other somatoform disorders, obscuring distinction (Hiller et al. 2000). For example, certain pain disorders—central pain states and fibromyalgia, for example—can mimic somatoform disorders. It is possible that a medical condition that is as yet unrecognized can lead, by default, to the erroneous conclusion that the pain associated with that condition is psychogenic. Patients with persisting pain, particularly pain with no clear etiology, might, as would the person with hypochondriasis, insist on finding a cause. This insistence might be grounded in the effort to convince the clinician of the legitimacy of the pain complaints and the need for treatment.

Somatic Amplification and Its Function

In some patients with pain, like patients with other somatoform disorders, amplification of somatic symptoms (including pain) may be a manifestation of psychological distress. For some persons, this amplification might reflect a strategy to cope with or manage psychological distress (Lipowski 1988). For others, somatic amplification may result from the distress associated with unpleasant affective states such as depression or anxiety. These emotional states may lead to heightened self-consciousness and a propensity to attend to bodily signals that might otherwise be ignored. Influenced by the distress of the prevailing emotional state combined with cognitive distortions (e.g., catastrophizing and magnification), as described in Chapter 3 ("Evaluation of the Pain

Table 4–3.   Psychiatric disorders in which pain can be a prominent complaint

Pain disorder
  Pain complaints the focus of clinical attention
  Associated psychological features (can be present or absent)
Somatization disorder
  At least four pain complaints
  Other somatic concerns (genitourinary or gastrointestinal)
  Pseudoneurologic disturbance
Hypochondriasis
  Preoccupation with fears of having a serious medical condition
  Based on a misinterpretation of bodily sensations, which can include discomfort
    or pain
Conversion disorder
  Loss of voluntary motor function or sensory function other than pain
Dyspareunia
  Pain arising exclusively during intercourse
Factitious disorder
  Deliberate deceit or feigning of symptoms (can include complaints of pain)
  No obvious secondary gain

Patient"; see Table 3–3), the individual is likely to misinterpret the bodily sensations as signaling a significant health- or pain-related disorder.

Somatic amplification can serve a number of psychological functions for the patient. For some patients, it can serve to secure and enlist the support of others. For other patients, it can serve to distance others or allow expression of discontent or anger or avoidance of interpersonal conflicts. In addition, some patients may derive benefits from the somatic amplification, such as avoidance of unpleasant tasks and responsibilities.

Somatic amplification and the focus on somatic symptoms can serve to mask other psychological symptoms. Depression in a patient presenting with somatic concerns is quite common. For example, for some patients, there might be the wish to deny depressive symptoms entirely, because to acknowledge them may incur the stigma of a psychiatric disorder or imply something about their character (e.g., weakness in the face of adversity). Still, for other patients, the propensity to present with somatic complaints may be based on

Table 4–4.   Factors that raise suspicion of malingering

Patient presentation to medical attention has a medicolegal context.

Marked discrepancy exists between patient's claims of disability or distress and objective findings.

Patient's reports may be vague, may be loaded with overgeneralizations, or may seem rehearsed. Patient history may fall apart when examiner's questions are reframed. Patient's responses to questions may be cryptic, and there is a tendency to hedge statements.

Once patient's objective is achieved, symptoms seem to take on less significance.

Patient rejects all forms of treatment that do not include psychoactive medications.

Patient exhibits lack of cooperation with medical diagnostic interventions.

Patient shows poor compliance with treatment interventions.

Antisocial personality disorder is present.

the belief that somatic concerns will be taken more seriously than will emotional factors (Lipowski 1990).

Pain and Deceit

Both factitious disorder and malingering involve the voluntary production or exaggeration of symptoms. Pain can be invoked with either condition. Although deceit is essential for both factitious disorder and malingering, the motives for the two conditions differ. In factitious disorder, the motive is to assume the "sick role"—that is, to gain something from the association with medical treatment; the motive does not include a concrete secondary gain. Malingerers, on the other hand, derive a clear secondary gain that could be understandable from the person's environmental circumstances. Examples of secondary gains include securing financial gain (e.g., from litigation or disability compensation), obtaining a haven (e.g., in the case of one who is homeless), and acquiring psychoactive substances (e.g., opiates). Factors that suggest possible malingering are summarized in Table 4–4.

Ailments claimed by patients seeking opiate analgesics typically include those not readily verifiable (e.g., renal colic, tic douloureux, sickle cell crisis). Thus, the patient might allege severe flank pain and provide a urine sample into which a drop of blood was deliberately placed. In the busy emergency department, such complaints can be met with a tendency to placate the patient with provision of the sought-out narcotic.

Depression

Among patients with chronic pain, depression prevalence rates were estimated at 30%–54%, much higher than in the general population (Banks and Kerns 1996). A number of studies have demonstrated that the severity of depressive symptoms predicted the number and severity of pain complaints (Dworkin et al. 1990; Faucett 1994). The causal relationships between depression and pain are unclear. Most data suggest that pain predisposes patients to depression (Fishbain et al. 1997) (i.e., developing as a consequence of pain [Gamsa 1990] or medical treatment [Massie and Holland 1990]). Alternatively, depression may precede the pain and may be related to its maintenance. In two longitudinal studies, depression predicted subsequent development of painful musculoskeletal disorders (Forseth et al. 1999; Leino and Magni 1993). The biopsychosocial approach to pain assessment recognizes that the relationship between pain and emotional disturbances (e.g., depression) is likely to be reciprocal.

Physiologic substrates common to both depression and pain are summarized in Table 4–5. Conceivably, a preexisting vulnerability (e.g., recurrent stress, preexisting depression) may increase the risk of developing chronic pain (diathesis) through modification of catecholamines and substance P and cytokine activity (Dersh et al. 2002). A perpetuating cycle is potentially set in motion such that with protracted pain and resultant increases in cytokine and substance P activity, the patient is predisposed to depression. The depression in turn can augment pain through cytokine activity, substance P activity, diminished opioid receptor responsiveness, and so on.

Patients with chronic pain are often plagued with distress related to unremitting pain, life changes, modifications in lifestyle and adaptive functioning, loss of rewarding activities, and a decline in social reinforcements. The potential pitfall is that clinicians might assume the depression is expected given the pain and overlook a potentially treatable disorder. Conversely, depression may be assumed to be present when physical examination and diagnostic interventions fail to account for the severity of the pain or if treatment measures are unsuccessful in mitigating pain. In such cases, the clinician can be misled into ignoring the pain complaints in the attempt to address the presumed depression. The patient may well construe this lack of attention to the pain complaints as devaluing the pain, causing confrontations to arise and possibly thwarting treatment measures.

Table 4–5. Physiologic substrates common to pain and depression

Physiologic substrate	Pain	Depression	Relationship
Catecholamines	Rostral ventromedial medulla (5-HT) and dorsolateral pontine tegmentum (NE) inhibit pain transmission from spinal dorsal horn.[a]	Locus coeruleus (NE) and raphe nucleus (5-HT) project to limbic system and other brain areas.[b]	Decreased catecholamines increase pain and depression.
Substance P	Binding to neurokinin receptors centrally and peripherally increases pain transmission.[c]	Central substance P activity is increased in animal paradigms of stress; inhibits activity of locus coeruleus and raphe nuclei.[d]	Increased central substance P activity increases pain and depression.
Opioid receptor	Modulate pain transmission centrally and peripherally.	Present in limbic structures; deactivation of μ-receptors is associated with dysphoria.[e]	Decreased activity can augment pain and depression.
Cytokines	Proinflammatory agents that promote pain.	Administration of interferon-alpha to patients induces depression.[f]	Increased activity augments pain and depression.

Note.   5-HT = serotonin; NE = norepinephrine.
[a]Fields and Basbaum 1999.
[b]Blier and Abbott 2001.
[c]Doyle and Hunt 1999.
[d]Mantyh 2002; Santarelli et al. 2002.
[e]Kennedy et al. 2006.
[f]Capuron et al. 2002.
Source.   Reprinted from Leo RJ: "Chronic Pain and Comorbid Depression." *Current Treatment Options in Neurology* 7:403–412, 2005. Copyright 2005, Current Science, Inc. Used with permission.

In assessing depression, the clinician should keep in mind that neuroveg-etative symptoms such as sleep disturbances, appetite changes, and fatigue can overlap considerably with symptoms of medical and surgical conditions asso-ciated with pain. Thus, reliance on these features may lead to the erroneous di-agnosis of a depressive disorder.

For effective diagnosis of depression in the medically ill, it may be best for the clinician to focus on the psychological symptoms of depression, which are un-likely to be influenced by medical conditions or their complications. Thus, loss of interests of any kind; lack of mood reactivity; lack of concentration; inde-cisiveness; and preoccupation with guilt, worthlessness, death, dying, suicide, despair, and hopelessness are more suggestive of an underlying depression (Cavanaugh 1984). Similarly, items in diagnostic scales—for example, the Beck Depression Inventory (Beck and Steer 1987)—can overlap considerably with medical symptoms, exaggerating depression severity in certain pain patients.

Anxiety

There is much speculation as to how anxiety can influence pain. For example, pain can heighten anxiety, which in turn can result in muscle strain and spasm. If the strain and spasm are severe enough, localized ischemia and muscle cell damage can arise, resulting in the release of pain-producing substances that then precipitate further pain. Heightened responses of lower back muscles, as shown by electromyography (EMG), were observed among patients discuss-ing personal anxiety-provoking stressors (Flor et al. 1985). Similarly, height-ened tension in frontal muscles, associated with personal distress, was noted among patients with tension headaches. This anxiety–pain relationship makes intuitive sense but has not been consistently borne out in evaluations using EMG. One reason for this is that although EMG can reflect activity in superfi-cial muscles, it may not measure the recordings of deeper muscles, where pain may actually originate. Also, a time lag is expected between the experience of distress and the production of muscle contraction and release of pain-producing substances (Flor and Turk 1989). If electromyographic recordings are not mea-sured for a sufficient duration to account for this lag time, it is conceivable that negative results would be yielded.

A general model of the anxiety–pain relationship is depicted in Figure 4–1. In this model, fear and apprehension precipitated by pain experiences may lead

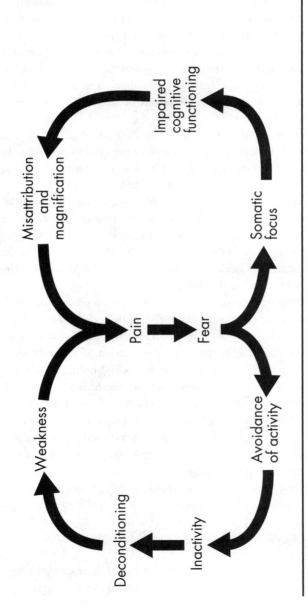

Figure 4–1. The anxiety–pain relationship.

to heightened somatic vigilance and concern. Anxiety over these experiences may give rise to cognitive distortions of physical symptoms, whose meaning may become distorted, magnified, and even amplified, leading to muscle tension and heightened pain. In addition, anxiety over precipitating pain can lead to restriction of movement and avoidance of physical therapy. This situation can further exacerbate pain by contributing to deconditioning and muscle weakness. Then, once activity is undertaken, one may be vulnerable to re-injury and pain (Asmundson et al. 1999).

Anxiety is common among patients with chronic pain. Anticipatory anxiety (e.g., preoperative anxiety) predicts increased rates of postoperative pain reporting and distress (Thomas et al. 1998). However, other researchers have questioned the impact of anxiety on pain states (Arntz et al. 1991). Anxiety disorders are accompanied by an increased incidence of somatic symptoms and pain complaints (Beidel et al. 1991). Anxious patients may experience higher than expected pain levels, mediated by limbic system activation. Limbic system activity during anxiety may nullify the pain-inhibiting processes that might normally emerge from the midbrain and descending inhibitory pathways (Merskey 1989), thereby intensifying the pain experience.

Patients with posttraumatic stress disorder (PTSD) often present with multiple physical ailments and complaints (McFarlane 1986). PTSD may accompany and perhaps exacerbate pain associated with traumatic injuries, warranting treatment. Patients with PTSD are prone to somatization, affective dysregulation, and dissociation. These patients lack the ability to differentiate between relevant and irrelevant information, predisposing them to focus attention on and misinterpret somatic experiences (van der Kolk et al. 1996).

Terminal cancer patients and others with chronic pain may experience existential anxiety, whereby a person questions the quality and meaning of life. Distress arises as one reflects on unaccomplished goals, time remaining to achieve goals, the meaning of one's life, one's legacy, and so on. The interruption of hoped-for life achievements can lead to marked dysphoria, anxiety, and narcissistic injury, requiring psychotherapy.

Sleep Disorders

Sleep disturbances frequently accompany pain. Patients often experience longer sleep onset latencies, frequent nighttime awakenings, and overall shorter duration of sleep (Morin et al. 1998). Such disturbances are likely to result from having a painful condition (e.g., rheumatoid arthritis, fibromyalgia, back pain) and would therefore be categorized as a sleep disorder due to a general medical condition according to DSM-IV-TR diagnostic criteria. However, it should be noted that sleep disturbances can reciprocally exacerbate pain severity. For example, deficits in Stage IV sleep, even among healthy individuals, may increase rates of reported muscle tenderness, aching, and stiffness (Moldofsky and Scarisbrick 1976). When these deficits are corrected, the painful symptoms often disappear.

Other factors (e.g., comorbid depression) may also contribute to sleep disturbances among patients with pain. Abnormalities in the sleep patterns of patients with fibromyalgia have been noted to likewise contribute to sleep disturbances. Specifically, alpha-delta sleep—in which intrusion of low-voltage, rapid alpha waves occurs amid higher voltage, slow waves characteristic of delta sleep—has been associated with fatigue and the perception that the sleep is nonrestorative (see also section "Fibromyalgia" in Chapter 8, "Common Pain Disorders," of this book). Additionally, patients with chronic pain (e.g., neuropathic conditions) may experience sleep difficulties secondary to restless legs syndrome (Yunus and Aldag 1996). Restless legs syndrome is characterized by tingling, paresthesias, and cramping (often of the lower extremities) that arises when one reclines but is transiently alleviated by movement. This need for movement interferes with sleep. Recognition of and differentiating among the possible etiologies for sleep disturbances of patients with pain is critical, as treatment approaches are partly defined by underlying causes. For example, an antidepressant may be warranted in cases of depression, whereas a dopamine agonist or anticonvulsant may be warranted to mitigate sleep difficulties arising from restless legs syndrome.

Substance-Related Disorders

The prevalence of substance dependence among patients with chronic pain is variable, ranging from 3.2% to 18.9% (Fishbain et al. 1992). The differences in the rates reported appear to be a result of the diagnostic criteria for dependence employed, the settings in which samples were gathered, and the types of chronic pain conditions examined. Although one study suggested that rates of substance dependence among patients with chronic pain and a comparable group of (nonpain) patients attending the same medical clinic did not differ significantly (Brown et al. 1996), further systematic investigation is warranted as to whether rates of substance dependence among patients with chronic pain differ from those in the general population.

Fear of drug addiction is often offered as an explanation of why clinicians have difficulty managing patients' pain. Such concerns are particularly heightened when treatment of chronic, nonmalignant pain is required. Patients with somatoform pain disorders may be more prone to dependence on psychoactive substances than patients with more serious physical illnesses (Streltzer et al. 2000). However, some studies indicate that among patients with chronic pain and substance use disorders, the substance use disorder preceded the onset of the pain disorder (Brown et al. 1996).

One feature of substance dependence suggestive of a pathologic state is the desire for acquisition of such substances (e.g., opiates) for something other than just pain relief (i.e., for psychological relief). Behaviors suggestive of substance abuse or dependence include problematic behaviors such as solicitation of medications from multiple sources, forgery of prescriptions, theft of medications, and acquisition of psychoactive substances from illegal sources.

Clinicians can be apt to misinterpret some behaviors of pain patients as being indicative of an underlying substance-related disorder. Referred to as *pseudoaddiction,* such behaviors are likely to arise when patients are undertreated (i.e., with inadequate dosage or inappropriately lengthy spacing of doses) with analgesics (Weissman and Haddox 1989). Deciphering between addiction and pseudoaddiction (see Table 4–6) can be somewhat difficult, however, and has been a source of controversy, in part because often no direct correlation can be found between objective medical findings or assessments and the degree of subjective pain complaints (Streltzer 2001; Streltzer et al. 2000). To acquire more analgesics, pseudoaddicted patients, like patients with substance dependence, may manipulate clinicians, embellish symptoms, and use up prescribed medications in excess of the intended rates. However, the agenda of pseudoaddicted patients, unlike the agenda of those with addiction, is based on a desire for pain relief. For pseudoaddicted patients, optimizing the analgesic treatment will eliminate future manipulative behaviors, whereas for addicted individuals it likely will not. Use of analgesics should enhance treatment adherence (e.g., participation in physical therapy) and improve adap-

Table 4–6.   Distinguishing features of pseudoaddiction and addiction

	Pseudoaddiction	Addiction
Dose escalation	Stops once pain is controlled	Continues
Goal	Pain relief	Euphoria/intoxication
Signs of intoxication	No	Yes
Concern over side effects	Yes	No
Follows other treatment suggestions	Yes	No
May invoke manipulative measures	Yes	Yes
Feigns symptoms	No	Yes
Withdrawal with abrupt cessation	Yes	Yes
Effect of provision of additional analgesic	Improved functioning	Worsened functioning

Source.   Adapted from Fishbain DA: "Chronic Pain and Addiction," in *Weiner's Pain Management: A Practical Guide for Clinicians,* 7th Edition. Edited by Boswell MV, Cole BE. Boca Raton, FL, CRC Taylor & Francis Press, 2006, p. 128. Copyright 2006, Routledge/Taylor & Francis Group. Used with permission.

tive functioning. If functioning improves once the analgesics are optimized, the presumption is that the behavior is indeed a reflection of an underlying pseudoaddiction. On the other hand, for the addicted patient, increased access to analgesics such as opiates will impair functioning.

Personality Disorders

Common personality disorders associated with chronic pain include histrionic, dependent, paranoid, and borderline types (Fishbain 1999). *Personality disorders* refers to long-standing, pervasive patterns of behavior, including patterns of relating to others, managing emotions, and viewing the world (reality testing). Diagnosis of such Axis II disorders should facilitate treatment, for example, by identifying those features of the personality that may interfere with treatment. Thus, the identification of a personality disorder should heighten the clinician's awareness of the patient's needs, the meanings of the illness to the patient, and the patient's coping repertoire (Weisberg and Keefe 1997). Unfortunately, for the patient with complex pain, the identification of Axis II disorders may be employed pejoratively to imply that the patient is difficult to treat and does little to facilitate or complement treatment.

One problem that frequently arises is whether the behaviors observed (those suggesting a personality disorder) are reflective of a long-standing pattern of functioning or whether they arise from the chronic pain experience. The patient may have a biological and environmental or developmental predisposition toward the expression of a particular personality trait characteristic of a disorder. Under ordinary circumstances, the predisposition might never be fully actualized. However, in a person who is under the stress of a chronic pain state—with its ensuing social, occupational, financial, and legal ramifications—such traits may be heightened and expressed in a manner that, on the surface, might suggest a personality disorder.

Schizophrenia

The literature on pain among patients with schizophrenia has suggested that these patients demonstrate an insensitivity or indifference to pain associated with serious medical conditions. A number of experimental paradigms have demonstrated that patients with schizophrenia tend to have reduced pain sensitivities and higher thresholds for pain compared with patients who do not have schizophrenia (Dworkin 1994). Reduced pain sensitivity was found to be a familial trait present among healthy relatives (i.e., without schizophrenia) of patients with schizophrenia (Hooley and Delgado 2001).

A number of mechanisms for these findings have been postulated. Higher pain thresholds have been correlated with higher levels of endogenous opioids in the cerebrospinal fluid in patients with schizophrenia as compared with those without schizophrenia. These endogenous opioids might mitigate awareness of and sensitivity to pain. In addition, alteration of cortical evoked potentials during noxious stimulation has been demonstrated, suggesting changes in the perception and processing of painful sensory information. Finally, disturbances in affective (limbic) systems accounting for the negative symptoms of schizophrenia may likewise interfere with the processing of pain and reactions to pain (Dworkin 1994).

Preliminary genetic studies have revealed that allelic variants of the δ-opiate receptor prevail among people with schizophrenia. The δ-receptor is normally responsive to endogenous opiates; however, the allelic variants observed among people with schizophrenia could be less sensitive to endogenous opiates (Xu et al. 2002). Thus, a feedback mechanism accounting for increased endogenous opiates in the cerebrospinal fluid might be explained. Further investigations are required to clarify the pathophysiology of pain insensitivity in schizophrenia.

Key Points

- To effectively manage most patients with chronic pain, clinicians must identify, diagnose, and treat common psychiatric comorbidities.
- The diagnosis of pain disorder assumes that pain is the primary symptom warranting clinical attention; the diagnostic taxonomy contained within DSM-IV-TR recognizes subtypes in the classification of pain disorder based on whether psychological factors contribute significantly to the pain experience.
- Critics of the diagnostic taxonomy of pain disorder in DSM-IV-TR contend that the criteria are insufficiently operationalized, failing to distinguish pain disorder from other psychiatric conditions, and that the nosology still retains vestiges of mind-body dualism.
- There are several common psychiatric comorbidities accompanying and complicating the experience of pain that warrant clinical attention and that can be the focus of psychiatric treatment. These include depression, anxiety, sleep disorders, somatoform disorders, substance-related disorders, and personality disorders.
- Expanding knowledge of the pathophysiology of pain processing and psychiatric disorders (e.g., depression) is beginning to unveil common neurologic substrates that may account for the high rates of co-occurrence of such conditions.
- Treating pain symptomatically without addressing psychiatric comorbidities is inadequate for the management of the patient, in part because it neglects potential sources of suffering and disability and potential impediments to the rehabilitation process.

References

Aigner M, Bach M: Clinical utility of DSM-IV pain disorder. Compr Psychiatry 40:353–357, 1999

American Psychiatric Association: Diagnostic and Statistical Manual of Mental Disorders, 3rd Edition. Washington, DC, American Psychiatric Association, 1980

American Psychiatric Association: Diagnostic and Statistical Manual of Mental Disorders, 3rd Edition, Revised. Washington, DC, American Psychiatric Association, 1987

American Psychiatric Association: Diagnostic and Statistical Manual of Mental Disorders, 4th Edition. Washington, DC, American Psychiatric Association, 1994

American Psychiatric Association: Diagnostic and Statistical Manual of Mental Disorders, 4th Edition, Text Revision. Washington, DC, American Psychiatric Association, 2000

Arntz A, Dreessen L, Merckelbach H: Attention, not anxiety, influences pain. Behav Res Ther 29:41–50, 1991

Asmundson GJG, Norton PJ, Norton GR: Beyond pain: the role of fear and avoidance in chronicity. Clin Psychol Rev 19:97–119, 1999

Banks SM, Kerns RD: Explaining high rates of depression in chronic pain: a diathesis-stress framework. Psychol Bull 119:95–110, 1996

Beck AT, Steer RA: Beck Depression Inventory Manual. San Antonio, TX, Psychological Corporation, 1987

Beidel DC, Christ MAG, Long PJ: Somatic complaints in anxious children. J Abnorm Child Psychol 19:659–670, 1991

Blier P, Abbott FV: Putative mechanisms of action of antidepressant drugs in affective and anxiety disorders and pain. J Psychiatry Neurosci 26:37–43, 2001

Brown RL, Patterson JJ, Rounds LA, et al: Substance abuse among patients with chronic back pain. J Fam Pract 43:152–160, 1996

Capuron L, Gumnick JF, Musselman DL, et al: Neurobehavioral effects of interferon-alpha in cancer patients: phenomenology and paroxetine responsiveness of symptom dimensions. Neuropsychopharmacology 26:643–652, 2002

Cavanaugh SVA: Diagnosing depression in the hospitalized patient with chronic medical illness. J Clin Psychiatry 45:13–16, 1984

Dersh J, Polatin PB, Gatchel RJ: Chronic pain and psychopathology: research findings and theoretical considerations. Psychosom Med 64:773–786, 2002

Doyle CA, Hunt SP: Substance P receptor (neurokinin-1)–expressing neurons in lamina I of the spinal cord encode for the intensity of noxious stimulation: a c-Fos study in rat. Neuroscience 89:17–28, 1999

Dworkin RH: Pain insensitivity in schizophrenia: a neglected phenomenon and some implications. Schizophr Bull 20:235–248, 1994

Dworkin RH, Caligor E: Psychiatric diagnosis and chronic pain: DSM-III-R and beyond. J Pain Symptom Manage 3:87–98, 1988

Dworkin SF, von Korff M, LeResche L: Multiple pains and psychiatric disturbance: an epidemiologic investigation. Arch Gen Psychiatry 47:239–244, 1990

Faucett JA: Depression in painful chronic disorders: the role of pain and conflict about pain. J Pain Symptom Manage 9:520–526, 1994

Fields HL, Basbaum AI: Central nervous system mechanisms of pain modulation, in Textbook of Pain, 4th Edition. Edited by Wall PD, Melzack R. Edinburgh, Scotland, Churchill Livingstone, 1999, pp 309–329

Fishbain DA: Approaches to treatment decisions for psychiatric comorbidity in the management of the chronic pain patient. Med Clin North Am 83:737–760, 1999

Fishbain DA: Chronic pain and addiction, in Weiner's Pain Management: A Practical Guide for Clinicians, 7th Edition. Edited by Boswell MV, Cole BE. Boca Raton, FL, CRC Taylor & Francis Press, 2006, pp 117–139

Fishbain DA, Goldberg M, Meagher BR, et al: Male and female chronic pain patients categorized by DSM-III psychiatric diagnostic criteria. Pain 26:181–197, 1986

Fishbain DA, Rosomoff HL, Rosomoff RS: Drug abuse, dependence, and addiction in chronic pain patients. Clin J Pain 8:77–85, 1992

Fishbain DA, Cutler R, Rosomoff HL, et al: Chronic pain–associated depression: antecedent or consequence of chronic pain? A review. Clin J Pain 13:116–137, 1997

Flor H, Turk DC: Psychophysiology of chronic pain: do chronic pain patients exhibit symptom-specific psychophysiologic responses? Psychol Bull 105:215–259, 1989

Flor H, Turk DC, Birbaumer N: Assessment of stress-related psychophysiological reactions in chronic back pain patients. J Consult Clin Psychol 53:354–364, 1985

Forseth KO, Husby G, Gran IT, et al: Prognostic factors for the development of fibromyalgia in women with self-reported musculoskeletal pain: a prospective study. J Rheumatol 26:2458–2467, 1999

Gamsa A: Is emotional disturbance a precipitator or a consequence of chronic pain? Pain 42:183–195, 1990

Hiller W, Heuser J, Fichter MM: The DSM-IV nosology of chronic pain: a comparison of pain disorder and multiple somatization syndrome. Eur J Pain 4:45–55, 2000

Hooley JM, Delgado ML: Pain insensitivity in the relatives of schizophrenic patients. Schizophr Res 47:265–273, 2001

Kennedy SE, Koeppe RA, Young EA, et al: Dysregulation of endogenous opioid emotion regulation circuitry in major depression in women. Arch Gen Psychiatry 63:1199–1208, 2006

Leino P, Magni G: Depressive and distress symptoms as predictors of low back pain, neck-shoulder pain, and other musculoskeletal morbidity: a 10-year follow-up of metal industry employees. Pain 53:89–94, 1993

Leo RJ: Chronic pain and comorbid depression. Curr Treat Options Neurol 7:403–412, 2005

Lipowski ZJ: Somatization: the concept and its clinical application. Am J Psychiatry 145:1358–1368, 1988

Lipowski ZJ: Somatization and depression. Psychosomatics 31:13–21, 1990

Mantyh PW: Neurobiology of substance P and the NK1 receptor. J Clin Psychiatry 63 (suppl 11):6–10, 2002

Massie MJ, Holland JC: Depression and the cancer patient. J Clin Psychiatry 51 (suppl 7):12–17, 1990

Mayou R, Levenson J, Sharpe M: Somatoform disorders in DSM-V. Psychosomatics 44:449–451, 2003

McFarlane AC: Posttraumatic morbidity of a disaster: a study of cases presenting for psychiatric treatment. J Nerv Ment Dis 174:4–14, 1986

Merskey H: Psychiatry and chronic pain. Can J Psychiatry 34:329–336, 1989

Moldofsky H, Scarisbrick P: Introduction of neurasthenic musculoskeletal pain syndrome by selective sleep stage deprivation. Psychosom Med 38:35–44, 1976

Morin CM, Gibson D, Wade J: Self-reported sleep and mood disturbance in chronic pain patients. Clin J Pain 14:311–314, 1998

Santarelli L, Gobbi G, Blier P, et al: Behavioral and physiologic effects of genetic or pharmacologic inactivation of the substance P receptor (NK1). J Clin Psychiatry 63 (suppl 11):11–17, 2002

Streltzer J: Pain management in the opioid-dependent patient. Curr Psychiatry Rep 3:489–496, 2001

Streltzer J, Eliashof BA, Kline AE, et al: Chronic pain disorder following physical injury. Psychosomatics 41:227–234, 2000

Sullivan MD: DSM-IV pain disorder: a case against the diagnosis. Int Rev Psychiatry 12:91–98, 2000

Thomas T, Robinson C, Champion D, et al: Prediction and assessment of the severity of post-operative pain and of satisfaction with management. Pain 75:177–185, 1998

van der Kolk BA, Pelcovitz D, Roth S, et al: Dissociation, somatization, and affect dysregulation: the complexity of adaptation to trauma. Am J Psychiatry 153:83–93, 1996

Weisberg JN, Keefe FJ: Personality disorders in the chronic pain population: basic concepts, empirical findings, and clinical implications. Pain Forum 6:1–9, 1997

Weissman DE, Haddox JD: Opioid pseudoaddiction: an iatrogenic syndrome. Pain 36:363–366, 1989

Xu J, Leo RJ, DiMartino S, et al: Linkage studies of delta opioid receptor gene and pain insensitivity in schizophrenia. Paper presented at the annual meeting of the American Psychiatric Association, Research Colloquium for Junior Investigators, Philadelphia, PA, May 2002

Yunus MB, Aldag JC: Restless legs syndrome and leg cramps in fibromyalgia syndrome: a controlled study. BMJ 312:1339, 1996

5

Pharmacology of Pain

Familiarity with the range of medications employed in the treatment of pain is essential. In this chapter I focus on the utility of such agents and the disorders in which they may be employed, as well as dosing and side effects.

Opiate Analgesics

Opiates have long been the mainstay of treatment in acute pain states and terminal disorders. However, long-term use in chronic, nonmalignant states has raised significant concerns for many clinicians about predisposing patients to functional impairments, dependence, and poor treatment response (Buckley et al. 1986; Finlayson et al. 1986; McNairy et al. 1984). Knowledge of opiate activity in the management of pain is essential. Familiarity with the dosing and duration of effects is required, as well as a knowledge of the ceiling effects (i.e., the maximal dose beyond which no further analgesic effect would be obtained) (Inturrisi 1984) (see Table 5–1).

Table 5–1. Opiate dosing and use

Agent	Equianalgesic dose, mg		Starting dose, mg	Duration, hours	Affinity for μ-receptor	Ceiling effect
	Oral	Parenteral				
Morphine-like agents						
Morphine	30	10	15–30 (oral)	4–5	+++	No
Codeine	200	120	30–60 (oral)	4–6	+	Yes
Hydromorphone	7.5	1.5	4–8 (oral)	4–5	+++	No
Meperidine	300	75	50–100[a] (oral)	2–5	++	No
Oxycodone	20	NA	15–30 (oral)	4–6[b]	++	No
Methadone	20	10	5–10 (oral)	3–8	+++	No
Levorphanol	4	2	2–4 (oral)	4–5	+++	No
Fentanyl[c]	—	0.1	0.1 (iv)	4–6	++++	No
Partial agonist						
Buprenorphine	—	0.4	0.3–0.6 (iv)	4–6	Partial	Yes

Table 5–1. Opiate dosing and use *(continued)*

Agent	Equianalgesic dose, mg		Starting dose, mg	Duration, hours	Affinity for μ-receptor	Ceiling effect
	Oral	Parenteral				
Agonist-antagonists						
Nalbuphine	—	10	10–20 (iv)	3–6	Antagonist	Yes
Butorphanol	—	2	0.5–2 (iv)	3–4	Antagonist	Yes
Dezocine	—	10	5–20 (iv)	3–6	Antagonist	Yes
Pentazocine	—	30	30–60 (iv)	3–4	Antagonist	Yes

Note. Dash (—) indicates not available in oral form. iv=intravenous; NA=not applicable.
[a]Higher starting doses may be required for moderate to severe pain.
[b]Sustained-release form available.
[c]Fentanyl transdermal patch not listed here.
Source. Bouckoms 1988; Cassem 1989; Jaffe and Martin 1990; Wise and Rundell 2005.

Table 5–2.   Medication suggestions for pain in the adult patient

Pain level	Medication suggestions
Mild (score of 1–3)	Acetaminophen, COX-2 inhibitor, NSAIDs, salicylates
Moderate (score of 4–6)	Codeine 30 mg with acetaminophen Hydrocodone 5 mg with acetaminophen Oxycodone 5 mg with acetylsalicylic acid (aspirin) or acetaminophen Tramadol 50 mg Tramadol 37.5 mg/acetaminophen 325 mg
Severe (score of 7–10)	Codeine 30–60 mg po q 3–4 hours Fentanyl (transdermal) 25 μg/hour q 3 days Hydrocodone 5–10 mg po q 4–6 hours Hydromorphone 4–8 mg po q 3–4 hours Methadone 5–10 mg po q 6–12 hours Morphine 15–30 mg po q 3–4 hours (immediate release or oral suspension) Oxycodone 10 mg po q 4–6 hours

Note.   COX-2= cyclooxygenase-2; NSAID=nonsteroidal anti-inflammatory drug. Suggestions here assume that pain scores are based on use of a numeric rating scale (see Chapter 3, "Evaluation of the Pain Patient," of this manual). In recommending these doses, it is assumed that patients are opiate naive; patients with prior opioid treatment use or opiate (e.g., heroin) dependence may require higher starting doses for optimal pain relief. Use morphine cautiously in patients with renal disease; hydromorphone may be preferred in such cases. Use acetaminophen cautiously; the maximum dose is 4,000 mg per 24 hours.

Guidelines for Use

The affinity of the opiates for the μ-receptors within the central nervous system (CNS) determines their effectiveness in mitigating pain. Certain opiates, such as codeine and propoxyphene, are considered to be weak opiates, useful in mild to moderate pain. For more severe pain, stronger opiates, such as morphine, are required. (General recommendations for mild, moderate, and severe pain are summarized in Table 5–2.)

Morphine is the agent against which all other opioids tend to be compared. Fentanyl is a very potent analgesic that has greater affinity for the μ-receptor than has morphine. The doses recommended in Tables 5–1 and 5–2 are offered as a guideline; the optimal analgesic dose may vary widely among patients. Opiate rotation—that is, sequential trials of analgesic—may be required to iden-

Table 5–3. Opioid therapy guidelines for chronic nonmalignant pain

Consider opiates after other reasonable alternatives have failed.

Consider contraindications for opiate use.

Prescription of opiates should be managed by a single practitioner.

Select opiates based on the following:

    Ease of administration (oral, transdermal, other)

    Cost

    Duration of analgesic effect

    Tolerability of side effects

    Potential risk of drug interactions

Administer opiates around the clock, instead of as needed.

Adjust or increase opiate dose gradually, contingent on the following:

    Degree of pain relief

    Degree of functional improvement

    Side-effect profiles

Address side effects.

Formalize treatment and document well.

Consider use of patient contract.

Consider making opiate therapy contingent on participation in other aspects of treatment (e.g., physical therapy, occupational therapy, psychotherapy).

Follow up weekly to monthly until patient is stable; once the patient is stabilized, less frequent follow-up may be possible.

tify the opiate that optimally addresses pain while offering the most favorably tolerated side effects. Equianalgesic doses of opiates must be a consideration. Selection of an opiate may be based on several factors (Table 5–3), including potential for medication side effects, drug interactions, complications related to medical comorbidities, and selection of optimal routes of medication administration (summarized later in this section).

Side Effects

The patient's prior experiences (efficacy of a drug or its untoward effects) might influence the clinician's analgesic choice. Affinity for the μ-receptor also determines the severity of the side effects encountered with opioids, influencing respiratory rate, gastrointestinal (GI) motility, sphincter tone, and so forth.

Side effects of opiate analgesics may include constipation, nausea, vomiting, excess sedation, pruritus, and respiratory depression. Laxatives may be used for constipation, and stimulants may be used for excessive sedation. Pruritus may be addressed with concomitant use of antihistamines (e.g., hydroxyzine). Respiratory depression is rare in patients who receive chronic opiate treatment, but it may arise with excessive doses and in opiate-naive patients. Reversal of respiratory depression may require the use of low doses of an opiate antagonist (e.g., naloxone). If opiate antagonists are used judiciously, it is possible to avoid precipitating pain or significant withdrawal symptoms.

To avoid some of the side effects associated with morphine-like opioids, a mixed agonist-antagonist is sometimes prescribed. The agonist-antagonist class of opioids consists of pentazocine, butorphanol, nalbuphine, and dezocine. These agents are agonists at κ-receptors but antagonists at μ-receptors, and they have less influence on the μ-receptors of the GI tract, producing less nausea, vomiting, and constipation than pure opiate agonists. Because these agents have antagonist properties, employing higher doses may actually depress analgesia. Ceiling effects limit the utility of such agents among certain patients.

Drug Interactions

Choice of opiate analgesic might be determined by other concurrently administered medications. Toxic reactions occur when meperidine is administered to patients taking monoamine oxidase inhibitors (MAOIs). When these medications are coadministered, a serotonin syndrome may result, producing diaphoresis, rigidity, hyperreflexia, hypertension or hypotension, tachycardia, delirium, seizures, hyperthermia, and occasionally death (Gratz and Simpson 1993; Sternbach 1991). More selective MAOIs—for example, selegiline, a monoamine oxidase B inhibitor used to treat parkinsonism and depression (e.g., selegiline transdermal)—may also interact with narcotic analgesics to produce toxic reactions. To avoid toxicity, the MAOI should be discontinued approximately 2 weeks before anticipated opiate initiation. When this is not possible, codeine, oxycodone, and morphine might be safer alternatives. Additionally, because the analgesic effects of the opiates may be potentiated by the interference of the hepatic metabolism caused by the MAOIs, the doses of opiates should be substantially lower than usual.

The analgesic effects of the opioids may be augmented by coadministration of several other psychotropic medications, including fluoxetine, tricyclic antidepressants (TCAs; e.g., amitriptyline, imipramine, clomipramine), and antipsychotics (e.g., promethazine, chlorpromazine, haloperidol) (Keeri-Szanto 1974; Maltbie et al. 1979; Stambaugh and Wainer 1981). To avoid untoward effects, lower opiate doses may be required if the opiate is coadministered with these agents. Opioids (e.g., propoxyphene) may inhibit the metabolism of TCAs (e.g., doxepin), leading to marked sedation and anticholinergic and α-adrenergic effects (Abernethy et al. 1982). Cigarette smoking diminishes the effectiveness of opiate analgesics (e.g., propoxyphene, pentazocine) by potentiating their metabolism.

Medical Conditions

Concurrent medical conditions might influence opiate selection. Among patients with renal failure, metabolites of selected opiates (i.e., morphine, meperidine, and propoxyphene) may produce significant untoward effects. The metabolites of these agents, which depend on renal clearance, may accumulate, producing prolonged sedation. In the case of meperidine, seizures and CNS toxicity may arise, whereas with propoxyphene, cardiac conduction abnormalities may develop. Doses of these agents must be reduced significantly in patients with renal compromise. Alternatively, hydromorphone lacks metabolites with significant activity and is a safer choice.

Route of Administration

The selected route of administration of the analgesic may be influenced by several factors, including ease of administration, degree of desired patient control, and tolerability of or preference for the administration route. The oral route of administration is convenient, flexible, and nonintrusive. The drawback of this route is that for most opiates, 1.5–2 hours must be allowed for peak drug effects. If patients have difficulty swallowing pills, liquid formulations are available. Some agents (e.g., hydromorphone) may be crushed and added to liquids for ingestion. For patients who are too incapacitated to swallow oral medications, alternative routes (e.g., transmucosal, transdermal, intramuscular, subcutaneous, intravenous, intraspinal) would have to be explored. Oral transmucosal fentanyl citrate is available. This formulation allows for rapid absorption of fentanyl for rapid pain relief (in 5–10 minutes) and is useful for patients with breakthrough pain despite optimal analgesic treatment. The peak analgesic effect with intramuscular administration has a faster onset but also dissipates faster than with oral administration; however, intramuscular administration is intrusive and painful. Repeated intramuscular opioid administration may lead to abscess formation and muscle fibrosis. Subcutaneous administration is an alternative to intramuscular injections and may be better tolerated. Intravenous administration of opiates is less intrusive, convenient, and quick acting. One variant of the intravenous infusion is patient-controlled analgesia (PCA), whereby the patient self-administers the drug and regulates administration (Table 5–4). When patients control the rate of opiate administration, they often require smaller doses of opiate than when they have to rely on dosing prescribed on an as-needed basis.

Transdermal fentanyl is slowly released through a reservoir, transfers through subcutaneous tissue, accumulates in subcutaneous fat tissue, and slowly diffuses into the bloodstream. A slow concentration gradient develops between the fat and neighboring blood vessels. Normally, fentanyl has a 3-hour half-life, but with the slow release from the subcutaneous reservoir, the effective half-life increases to 17 hours. Because of the delay in movement to the bloodstream, transdermal fentanyl will not have immediate analgesic effects for approximately the first 24 hours. Consequently, during this time, supplemental analgesics are required. Once the effectiveness of the fentanyl patch has been appreciated, the supplemental analgesics may be discontinued. The patch needs to be replaced every 3 days. Both PCA and transdermal administration offer the advantage of reduced demand on staff time for administering as-needed opiates.

In some cases, switching from one route to another may require significant dose modifications. For example, oral meperidine has approximately one-fourth the analgesic efficacy of similar parenteral doses. Thus, when a switch from intramuscular to oral meperidine is made, four times the parenteral dose is generally required.

Continuous pain, present most of the day, requires that analgesics be administered around the clock as opposed to being administered as needed (Portenoy and Hagen 1990). When medications are dispensed as needed, higher doses of the opiate may be required to relieve pain. Furthermore, a longer period of time might elapse before sufficient relief is attained. Scheduled analgesics might avoid both of these difficulties.

When treated with short-acting agents (see Table 5–1), patients may experience recurrence of pain at the end of the dosing interval, when levels of the

Table 5–4. Dosing guidelines

1. Converting from conventional immediate-release oral morphine (or equivalent) to controlled-release morphine

   a. Calculate the total amount of conventional immediate-release oral morphine (or equivalent) used in a 24-hour period.

   b. Divide this amount by 3.

   c. The resulting amount is the dose of controlled-release morphine to be administered three times daily.

2. Converting from oral morphine (or equivalent) to transdermal fentanyl

   a. Calculate the total amount of oral morphine (or equivalent) employed in a 24-hour period.

   b. Divide total oral morphine dose by 3.

   c. Select the nearest patch strength in µg/hour (i.e., 25, 50, 75, or 100 µg/hour).

   d. Continue to administer the scheduled oral morphine for the first 12–24 hours after the first patch is in place.

3. Converting from oxycodone to extended-release oxycontin

   a. Calculate the total amount of oral oxycodone employed in a 24-hour period.

   b. Divide the total oxycodone dose by 2.

   c. The resulting amount is the dose of extended-release oxycontin to be administered twice daily.

4. PCA specifications

   a. Administer loading dose, generally 1–2 mg of morphine (or equivalent).

   b. Decide the hourly rate of the opiate that will be administered continuously (e.g., 1–2 mg morphine [or equivalent] hourly).

   The patient-requested rate needs to be determined. The PCA has lockout periods, during which no opiate will be administered even if the patient presses the button to administer the medication. The lockout period is generally determined to be 6–12 minutes. The patient will be able to self-administer 1–2 mg morphine (or equivalent) when the button is pressed beyond the preestablished lockout period.

Note. PCA = patient-controlled analgesia.

analgesic agent are reduced. Such effects, including interference with sleep, may be difficult for patients to tolerate. Longer-acting agents, therefore, are preferred. With these agents, pain recrudescence at the end of the dosing interval is less likely to occur. Agents such as levorphanol have long durations of action, as compared with morphine, and might be useful in this regard. Longer-acting formulations of other agents (e.g., controlled-released morphine, controlled-release oxycodone, transdermal fentanyl) are now available for sustained analgesia (see Table 5–4). Such formulations allow for more gradual release through the GI tract and may be dosed at 6- and 12-hour intervals. Crushing of the slow-release formulations (e.g., to be administered via nasogastric tube) will result in release of all of the opioid and eliminates any long-acting effects.

As with transdermal fentanyl, long-acting formulations do not produce immediate relief. Thus, supplementation with short-acting agents may be required until the analgesic effects of the long-acting agent are appreciated.

Agents With Multiple Uses

Methadone has been used primarily for opioid detoxification and maintenance treatment of individuals with opioid dependence. Its utility in such situations is that it has a long half-life and binds preferentially to opiate receptors. Methadone has analgesic ability as well. Its analgesic effects are short-lived, however; thus, more frequent dosing is required. For patients already receiving methadone maintenance therapy, their usual doses may be divided to optimize pain relief. Patients requiring methadone maintenance acquire the drug on an outpatient basis by appearing at the methadone clinics daily. If a patient were to simultaneously require pain management—that is, more frequent dosing with smaller doses—the patient would have to appear at the clinic several times daily, which could prove to be logistically difficult. A federal license is required to prescribe methadone for detoxification or maintenance treatment related to opioids but is not required for purposes of pain management.

Methadone is available in two isomeric forms, the *d-* and *l-*isomers. Although the *d-*isomer does not bind to the opiate receptor, it does bind to *N*-methyl-D-aspartate (NMDA) receptors. It is thought that this action may exert an analgesic effect independent of μ-receptor binding. Thus, the methadone is likely to be more potent than expected by conventional opiate pharmacokinetics. When switching patients from one opiate to methadone, some clinicians advocate a reduction of as much as 75%–90% in the dose because of the unexpectedly high potency of the methadone.

Buprenorphine is a partial agonist that binds preferentially to μ-receptors and has antagonist activities at the κ-receptors. Its effects (e.g., respiratory depression) are not easily reversed by antagonists (e.g., naloxone). It is administered intravenously for pain control in moderate to severe pain. There is an analgesic ceiling effect; thus, for pain persisting beyond optimal dosing, the clinician may have to explore alternatives. Buprenorphine is approved by the U.S. Food and Drug Administration (FDA) for the treatment of opioid dependence. It is administered sublingually for this purpose, either alone or in combination with naloxone.

Tolerance, Dependence, and Pseudoaddiction

Tolerance may emerge with the long-term use of opiate analgesics—that is, higher doses are required to achieve the same level of analgesia previously achieved at lower doses. Because of this propensity, opiate rotation has been advocated. To rotate from one opiate analgesic to another, refer to the equianalgesic doses shown in Table 5–1. Because the cross-tolerance among opioids is incomplete, the equianalgesic dose of the newer agent is reduced by 25%–50% of its usual prescribed dose. Alternatively, supplementation with adjunctive agents (e.g., nonopioid analgesics) may augment the analgesic effect of the opiate without requiring significant opiate dose increments.

If a patient presents with increases in pain despite analgesic use, it is inappropriate to assume that this increase reflects tolerance without first examining the patient and determining if another health condition has emerged that warrants attention. It is possible that disease progression or a secondary illness or physical process is emerging, aggravating the pain despite analgesic use and requiring alternative treatment interventions (Portenoy 1996).

A common misconception is that the development of tolerance might signal dependence. Physical dependence is probable with the long-term use of opiate analgesics. It is likely present if the patient develops signs of opiate withdrawal when the dosage is suddenly reduced or the agent is abruptly discontinued. Signs may include lacrimation, rhinorrhea, gooseflesh, irritability and anxiety, nausea, vomiting, abdominal cramping, lower extremity cramping, and other features. If the opioid needs to be discontinued after long-term use, the process should be undertaken gradually to avoid the unnecessary discomfort that accompanies abrupt withdrawal. Because of their antagonist properties, the clinician must be cautious about administering agonist-antagonists to patients with opiate dependence or to those previously treated with full agonist opiates. Agonist-antagonists may likewise precipitate withdrawal, adding significant distress to the pain already experienced. Alternatively, methadone may be employed to successfully detoxify the patient while minimizing withdrawal symptoms. Use of adjunctive agents (e.g., transdermal clonidine) may also reduce some of the autonomic symptoms that may accompany withdrawal.

Patients who are inadequately treated with opiate analgesics may display behaviors (i.e., pseudoaddiction) that on the surface appear to be manipulative and characteristic of drug seeking (Weissman and Haddox 1989). These behaviors generally cease once opioids are dosed appropriately to mitigate pain. However, distinguishing substance dependence from pseudoaddiction may be difficult (see the section "Substance-Related Disorders" in Chapter 4, "Common Psychiatric Comorbidities and Psychiatric Differential Diagnosis of the Pain Patient," of this book).

Clinicians may be uncomfortable about prescribing opioids for the long term, especially in cases of chronic nonmalignant pain, because of concerns about federal regulations and the risks of substance abuse. To ease their concern, they may establish a patient contract (see also Table 10–1 in Chapter 10, "Forensic Issues Pertaining to Pain,"of this book).

Tramadol

Tramadol is unique in its pharmacologic effects. It has opiate effects (affinity for the μ-receptor is approximately one-tenth that of codeine) and influences other neurotransmitter pathways (i.e., it inhibits the reuptake of norepinephrine [NE] and serotonin [5-HT]). Both NE and 5-HT are thought to inhibit the influence of pain-mediating neurotransmitters (i.e., substance P) within the dorsal horn of the spinal cord. A newer variant combining the anti-inflammatory effects of acetaminophen (325 mg) with tramadol (37.5 mg) (i.e., Ultracet), as well as a once-daily tramadol extended-release formulation, is available.

Tramadol use has been associated with seizures, although the risk is low; the risk may, however, increase with concomitant antidepressant (e.g., bupropion) use. In addition, serotonin syndrome may result from combinations of tramadol with selective serotonin reuptake inhibitors (SSRIs).

The abuse and dependence liability of tramadol was once thought to be quite low. However, several reports have emerged that indicate that tramadol is an agent on which patients may become quite dependent. In one case, a patient had been using such dramatic daily amounts that inpatient methadone detoxification was required (Leo et al. 2000).

Nonopiate Analgesics

Acetylsalicylic acid (aspirin), other salicylates, acetaminophen, nonsteroidal anti-inflammatory drugs (NSAIDs), and cyclooxygenase-2 (COX-2) inhibitors are useful for treating acute and chronic pain. These nonopioid agents act by interfering with prostaglandin synthesis and disrupting pain by reducing inflammation at peripheral sites. (However, the mechanism of the analgesia produced by acetaminophen is unclear.) Some of these are also useful as antipyretic agents. The efficacy of these agents is limited by a ceiling effect, and their usefulness is limited by the risk of side effects.

Aspirin produces irreversible platelet aggregation, a concern if surgery is anticipated in the near future. Other salicylates (e.g., choline magnesium trisalicylate, salsalate) have fewer GI side effects and less effect on bleeding time. Reye's syndrome is associated with aspirin use in children who have a viral illness (varicella). Aspirin hypersensitivity is of two types: one involving respiratory reactions (observed in patients with rhinitis, asthma, or nasal polyps), and the second involving rapid development of urticaria, angioedema, hypotension, shock, or syncope.

Acetaminophen does not produce GI distress, nor does it produce platelet inhibition. However, when combined with warfarin, it may predispose patients to marked anticoagulation and bleeding. Severe hepatotoxicity may arise with excessive use of acetaminophen and with concurrent use of alcohol and acetaminophen. Patients should therefore restrict their alcohol use when taking acetaminophen.

NSAIDs have efficacy comparable to that of the salicylates and are viable alternatives for persons with hypersensitivities to aspirin. However, there are occasional cross-sensitivities to NSAIDs in aspirin-sensitive individuals. Some NSAIDs have significantly more analgesic efficacy than salicylates (e.g., parenteral ketorolac has analgesic efficacy comparable to that of 6–12 mg of morphine). NSAIDs are nonselective inhibitors of the cyclooxygenase enzyme responsible for the prostaglandin synthesis in peripheral tissues that results in inflammatory pain. Because of their lack of selectivity, NSAIDs have inhibitory effects on the COX-1 enzyme, interfering with prostaglandins that mediate beneficial physiologic effects in the GI tract and renal tubules.

The most problematic side effects of NSAID use are gastric irritation and ulceration, bleeding due to reduced platelet aggregation, and renal dysfunction. Unlike aspirin, NSAIDs do not produce irreversible platelet inhibition. Patients at risk for GI disturbances are those of advanced age, those with histories of prior ulcers, and those simultaneously receiving steroids. To reduce the risk of GI complications, the lowest doses possible should be used. Use of misoprostol or omeprazole may be efficacious in preventing ulcers. Ranitidine and cimetidine are not useful in preventing ulceration, but they may be employed to treat the gastric ulcers produced by NSAID use. NSAIDs may reduce renal blood flow and glomerular filtration. As a consequence, there is increased water and electrolyte reabsorption in the proximal tubule, predisposing vulnerable persons to increased blood pressure and congestive heart failure. Other toxic effects of NSAIDs include hepatotoxicity and acute renal failure.

The use of NSAIDs has been associated with the emergence of psychiatric disturbances (e.g., depression, paranoia) among older patients. Although the mechanisms underlying this association are unclear, blockade of prostaglandin synthesis may be related to alterations in modulation of 5-HT and dopamine neurotransmitter systems within the CNS. The influence of NSAIDs on psychiatric symptoms is suggested by the close temporal relationship between drug initiation and onset of symptoms; this effect may occur in individuals with and without preexisting psychiatric illness (Browning 1996; Jiang and Chang 1999). Concomitant use of NSAIDs and lithium may lead to lithium toxicity. Aspirin, acetaminophen, and perhaps the NSAID sulindac may be safely employed in patients concomitantly treated with lithium (Ragheb and Powell 1986).

Cyclooxygenase-2 Inhibitors

COX-2 inhibitors, because of their selectivity, are less likely than NSAIDs to produce any adverse GI or renal effects. Only celecoxib is currently available for use in the United States; rofecoxib and valdecoxib were removed from the market because of adverse effects. Celecoxib (100 mg twice daily) has been useful in reducing pain associated with osteoarthritis; a dosage of 200 mg twice daily has been employed to manage rheumatoid arthritis and sickle cell pain.

Concerns have been raised regarding the cardiovascular safety of the COX-2 inhibitors. The alleged mechanism underlying the risk for adverse cardiovascular events is thought to be related to the prothrombotic effects of the COX-2 inhibitors. Specifically, by interfering with the COX-2 enzyme, these agents interfere with prostacyclin formation, which confers beneficial vascular effects. Because these agents do not block the COX-1 enzyme, the formation of thromboxane A_2 goes unchecked (see Figure 5–1). The latter confers prothrombotic effects, predisposing patients to potential risks of myocardial infarction, ischemic stroke, pulmonary embolism, and so on.

As a result, use of COX-2 inhibitors should be avoided in patients with risk factors for cardiovascular events (e.g., hypertension, hyperlipidemia, diabetes mellitus, cigarette smoking). Use is contraindicated in patients with congestive heart failure, ischemic heart disease, cerebrovascular disease, or severe peripheral arterial disease, as well as patients with sensitivities to COX-2 inhibitors or allergies to sulfonamides or NSAIDs. Concomitant use of aspirin, although it reduces risk of cardiovascular complications, may increase GI complications that would otherwise have been preventable with use of the COX-2 inhibitor.

Antidepressants

Antidepressants have long been advocated for the treatment of several chronic pain disorders. Pain reduction with use of antidepressants has been demonstrated among nondepressed pain patients. Among depressed pain patients, antidepressants may produce analgesia faster and at doses far lower than those required for antidepressant effects.

The pain-mitigating effects of antidepressants remain a subject of intensive investigation and are thought to involve a number of supraspinal, spinal, and peripheral processes (see Table 5–5). Analgesia produced by antidepressants is thought to be primarily mediated by enhancement of the inhibitory neurotransmitters (e.g., NE and 5-HT) present within descending pain-mediating pathways. In the spinal cord, the synthesis and release of pain-promoting neurotransmitters (e.g., glutamate) are reduced by these agents. In addition, certain antidepressants may augment opiate effects within the spinal cord. Morphine analgesia is potentiated by amitriptyline, imipramine, clomipramine, fluoxetine, sertraline, and nefazodone (Larson and Takemori 1977; Lee and Spencer 1980; Pick et al. 1992; Taiwo et al. 1985). On the other hand, within the brain, the antidepressants reduce the extent of limbic output, which might otherwise contribute to depression and anxiety that exacerbate underlying pain.

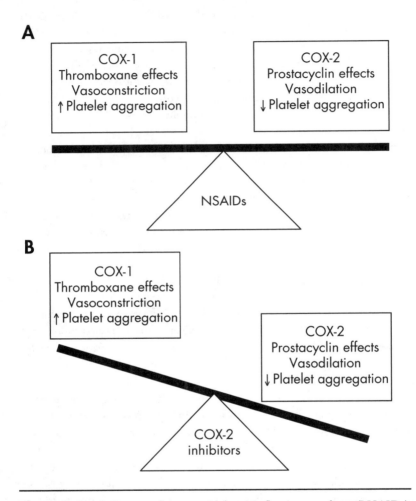

Figure 5–1.   Influence of nonsteroidal anti-inflammatory drugs (NSAIDs) and cyclooxygenase-2 (COX-2) inhibitors on thromboxane and prostacyclin effects.

(A) NSAIDs, by blocking thromboxane and prostacyclin effects simultaneously, keep both prothrombotic and antithrombotic effects in balance, without significantly altering the patients' risk of cardiovascular events. (B) COX-2 inhibitors, by blocking prostacyclin, leave the thromboxane effects unabated, predisposing patients to vasoconstriction and platelet aggregation, increasing the risk of cardiovascular events.

Tricyclic Antidepressants

The bulk of the evidence pertaining to the use of antidepressants in pain states has been directed at the utility of TCAs (Table 5–6). Neuropathic and idiopathic pains may respond better to TCA use than do nociceptive pains. However, these agents may be effective in nociceptive pain states when there is a comorbid depression or anxiety that complicates the disorder. The efficacy of TCAs appears to be related to the reuptake inhibition of NE and 5-HT. TCAs with a broad spectrum of activity may be more effective in pain reduction than those with neurotransmitter-specific effects. Thus, amitriptyline and imipramine appear to be more effective than desipramine or clomipramine (Max et al. 1992).

Generally speaking, TCAs are initiated at a dose of 10–25 mg at bedtime. Analgesia appears to be dose dependent. The dose may be increased slowly (e.g., increased in increments of 10–25 mg every 3–7 days) until analgesia or intolerable side effects occur. Specific analgesic serum levels for the TCAs are unknown. However, if a dosage of 150 mg/day is achieved without significant pain relief, assessment of serum levels may be prudent. This assessment may help to ascertain whether there is poor adherence to the medication regimen, poor absorption, rapid metabolism of the TCA, or all of these factors. If the patient is adherent to the regimen but, because of metabolic factors, has seemingly low serum levels, the dosage of the TCA may be increased beyond 150 mg/day if the side effects are not prohibitive. Serum levels should be checked to assess for toxic ranges, particularly for nortriptyline. However, if side effects preclude dose advancement, alternatives need to be considered.

Unfortunately, the adverse effects of the TCAs may limit their utility (Table 5–7). Amitriptyline and imipramine have more troublesome side effects than the secondary-amine TCAs (e.g., nortriptyline and desipramine). TCAs are contraindicated in patients with closed-angle glaucoma, recent myocardial infarction, cardiac arrhythmias, poorly controlled seizures, or severe benign prostatic hypertrophy.

Serotonin-Norepinephrine Reuptake Inhibitors

The serotonin-norepinephrine reuptake inhibitors (SNRIs) (i.e., venlafaxine and duloxetine) have demonstrated utility as analgesic agents, and they bypass several of the untoward effects commonly associated with the TCAs. Both agents have been demonstrated to have pain-mitigating effects in randomized con-

Table 5–5. Analgesic effects of antidepressants

Site of action		Mechanism	Effect
Supraspinal[a]	Descending inhibitory fibers from raphe nucleus and locus coeruleus	Increased 5-HT and NE	Enhanced pain modulation through heightened activity of descending fibers extending to the dorsal horn
Spinal	Pain-inhibitory interneurons[b]	Stimulation of α_1-adrenergic receptors	Increased GABA and glycine release, inhibiting pain transmission
	Pain-promoting interneurons[c]	Stimulation of α_2-adrenergic receptors	Decreased glutamate release, preventing further pain augmentation
Peripheral	Peripheral neurons[d]	Voltage-gated sodium channel blockade	Decreased firing of neurons, reduced input to the dorsal horn
	Inflammation[e]	5-HT_2 antagonism	Reduced pain in formalin models of pain

Note. 5-HT=serotonin; GABA=γ-aminobutyric acid; NE=norepinephrine.
[a]Sindrup and Jensen 1999; Fields and Basbaum 1999.
[b]Baba et al. 2000.
[c]Kawasaki et al. 2003.
[d]Gerner et al. 2001.
[e]Abbott et al. 1997.

Table 5–6. Antidepressants used in chronic pain

Tricyclic antidepressants	Monoamine oxidase	Trazodone
Neuropathy	inhibitors	Diabetic neuropathy
Diabetic type	Peripheral neuropathy	
Postherpetic	Migraine headache	**Nefazodone**
Poststroke		Headache
Nondiabetic peripheral	**Selective serotonin**	Tension
Headache	**reuptake inhibitors**	Migraine
Tension	Diabetic neuropathy	
Migraine	Tension headache	**Mirtazapine**
Rheumatologic disorders		Chronic daily tension
Fibromyalgia	**Serotonin-norepinephrine**	headache
Osteoarthritis	**reuptake inhibitors**	Fibromyalgia
Rheumatoid arthritis	Fibromyalgia	
Other	Chronic headache	
Atypical facial pain	Diabetic neuropathy	
Phantom limb pain	Peripheral neuropathy	
Complex regional pain		
syndrome	**Bupropion**	
	Peripheral neuropathy	

trolled trials of patients with neuropathy (Goldstein et al. 2005; Rowbotham et al. 2004; Sindrup et al. 2003) or fibromyalgia (Arnold et al. 2004; Zijlstra et al. 2002), with and without comorbid depression. Duloxetine has received FDA approval for treatment of diabetic neuropathy. Simultaneous NE and 5-HT influences are achieved at low doses with duloxetine; a dosage as low as 20 mg/day may be sufficient (Goldstein et al. 2005). For venlafaxine, unlike duloxetine, the 5-HT effects predominate at low doses. It may be necessary to dose at an antidepressant level to achieve pain-mitigating effects, (Zijlstra et al. 2002). Adverse effects of SNRIs may include nausea, dry mouth, nervousness, constipation, and somnolence. Venlafaxine may be associated with weight loss and elevations in diastolic blood pressure. If TCAs are not tolerated by the pain patient, these agents may prove to be workable alternatives.

Selective Serotonin Reuptake Inhibitors

SSRIs offer the advantages of greater tolerability of side effects and relative safety in overdose as compared with TCAs. However, the literature on SSRI effectiveness is limited by the small sample sizes and small dosage ranges employed in the

Table 5–7.   Tricyclic antidepressant side effects

Anticholinergic	Cardiac
Dry mouth	Palpitations
Constipation	Sweating
Memory impairments	Tachycardia
Blurred vision	Prolonged Q-T interval
Urinary retention	Neurologic
Delirium	Myoclonus
Antihistamine	Tardive dyskinesia
Sedation	Parkinsonism
Weight gain	Seizures
α-Adrenergic	
Orthostatic hypotension	

published studies (Ansari 2000). SSRIs found to be effective for one type of pain do not necessarily have efficacy in other types (e.g., fluoxetine may be useful for chronic daily tension headaches but might not be effective for diabetic neuropathy) (Diamond and Freitag 1989; Saper et al. 1994). Similarly, the effectiveness of one SSRI cannot be generalized to other SSRIs (i.e., if one SSRI is effective for a certain type of pain, this does not mean that other SSRIs will show similar efficacy). For example, paroxetine appears to be effective for neuropathic pain, but fluoxetine does not (Max et al. 1992; Sindrup et al. 1990, 1991).

There is some question whether the reduced efficacy of SSRIs as compared with TCAs is related to the 5-HT selectivity of SSRIs. As noted in the section on TCAs, those TCAs with broader spectra of neurotransmitter activity tend to be more effective than those with more selective 5-HT activity. In one study, fluoxetine was less effective than amitriptyline and desipramine and was no better than placebo (Max et al. 1992).

Doses of SSRIs are increased slowly as tolerated and as warranted by the need for analgesic, antidepressant, or anxiolytic efficacy. Side effects associated with their use include nausea, diarrhea, insomnia or sedation, tremors, and sexual dysfunction.

Other Antidepressants

Bupropion is an antidepressant with a broad spectrum of activity of neurotransmitters, including NE, 5-HT, and dopamine, and has displayed some promise with respect to efficacy in neuropathic pain (Semenchuk et al. 2001) (see Table 5–6). Bupropion lacks significant cardiac or anticholinergic side effects and has fewer risks of drug interactions; however, there is a risk of seizure associated with higher doses.

Mirtazapine may be helpful in mitigating symptoms associated with fibromyalgia (Samborski et al. 2004) and prophylaxis of chronic daily tension headache (Bendtsen and Jensen 2004). Researchers in two studies—one involving patients with neuropathy and the other involving chronic headache patients—found pain-mitigating effects with nefazodone. Patients with migraine or tension headache experienced marked reductions in the frequency, severity, and duration of recurrent headache when treated with daily nefazodone (Goodnick et al. 2000; Saper et al. 2001). Nefazodone use has been linked with hepatic dysfunction, and its use should be avoided in patients concurrently taking medications with potential hepatotoxic effects (e.g., acetaminophen). Additional clinical trials investigating the roles of these antidepressants are warranted.

Trazodone appears to be minimally, but not conclusively, efficacious in pain. Although two double-blind studies demonstrated efficacy of trazodone in diabetic neuropathy and pain resulting from nerve deafferentation (Khurana 1983; Ventafridda et al. 1988), the effects on patients with headache, fibromyalgia, rheumatoid arthritis, or chronic low back pain seemed less promising (Ansari 2000). Trazodone has been employed for its sedative properties. Some patients, particularly those taking opiates or other sedating agents, may find the sedative effects too incapacitating. The analgesic properties of trazodone appear to be independent of its sedative effects (Ansari 2000). Caution concerning other potential adverse effects associated with trazodone use (e.g., orthostasis, priapism) is warranted; doses should be kept to a minimum and increased only gradually to reduce the risk of incurring adverse effects.

The MAOI phenelzine has been found to be effective in the treatment of selected pain disorders. However, MAOI use has been limited by medication side effects, the need for a tyramine-free diet, and the potential risk of drug interactions (e.g., serotonin syndrome arising from coadministration with meperidine).

Although not currently available in the United States, emerging antidepressant therapies potentially useful for pain include milnacipran, an SNRI; and reboxetine, an NE reuptake inhibitor (Krell et al. 2005; Leo and Brooks 2006; Vitton et al. 2004). Milnacipran has demonstrated efficacy in the relief

Table 5–8.   Uses of anticonvulsants in various pain conditions

Carbamazepine	Oxcarbazepine
Trigeminal neuralgia	Trigeminal neuralgia
Neuropathy	Tiagabine
Gabapentin	Diabetic polyneuropathy
Neuropathy	Peripheral neuropathy
Atypical facial pain	Phantom limb pain
Reflex sympathetic dystrophy	Pregabalin
Central pain	Postherpetic neuralgia
Migraine prophylaxis	Diabetic neuropathy
Divalproex sodium	Phenytoin
Migraine prophylaxis	Trigeminal neuralgia
Neuropathy	Diabetic neuropathy
Lamotrigine	Topiramate
Trigeminal neuralgia	Neuropathy
Peripheral neuropathy	Migraine prophylaxis
Central neuropathy	

of pain associated with fibromyalgia; reboxetine has been used in case reports of patients with musculoskeletal pain and fibromyalgia.

Anticonvulsant Drugs

Anticonvulsant drugs (ACDs) historically have demonstrated efficacy in neuropathic pain, including trigeminal neuralgia and phantom limb pain (McQuay et al. 1995), as well as migraine (Pappagallo 2003; Snow et al. 2002) (Table 5–8). The mechanisms underlying analgesia produced by ACDs are varied (e.g., slowing the peripheral nerve conduction of primary afferent fibers and thereby dampening the painful sensory information relayed to the CNS, modulating sodium and/or calcium channel activity) (see Table 5–9). In addition, ACDs also function to inhibit the production of pain-promoting neurotransmitters (Swerdlow 1984).

Gabapentin has received FDA approval for use in the treatment of neuropathic pain. Gabapentin offers numerous advantages over other available ACDs. It is unlikely to produce serious side effects associated with the use of other anticonvulsants (e.g., hyponatremia associated with carbamazepine, hepatic effects associated with valproate). Patients taking gabapentin do not require

Table 5–9. Anticonvulsant mechanisms of action relevant to pain

Drug	Decrease in Na channel activity	Increase in CNS GABA activity	Modulation of Ca^{2+} channels	Reduction of EAA activity
Carbamazepine	+			
Phenytoin	+			
Valproate	+	+	+	
Gabapentin	+	+	+ (?)	
Lamotrigine	+		+	
Oxcarbazepine	+			
Topiramate	+	+		+
Pregabalin		+	+	
Tiagabine		+		
Zonisamide	+		+	

Note. Ca^{2+} = calcium; CNS = central nervous system; EAA = excitatory amino acid; GABA = γ-aminobutyric acid; Na = sodium.
Source. Adapted from Leo RJ: "Treatment Considerations in Neuropathic Pain." *Current Treatment Options in Neurology* 8:389–400, 2006. Copyright 2006, Current Science, Inc.; Massie MJ (ed.): *Pain: What Psychiatrists Need to Know* (Review of Psychiatry Series, Vol 19; Oldham JM and Riba MB, series eds.). Washington, DC, American Psychiatric Press, 2000, p. 37. Copyright 2000, American Psychiatric Press.

serum drug, hematologic, electrolyte, or hepatic enzyme monitoring, as is often required with other ACDs. The most common adverse events reported with its use are somnolence, dizziness, ataxia, tremor, fatigue, and nystagmus. Gabapentin is excreted unchanged from the kidneys; plasma clearance is proportional to creatinine clearance (McLean 1994). Dose reductions are required for patients with compromised renal functioning and those who require dialysis.

Pregabalin has been FDA approved for both postherpetic neuralgia and diabetic neuropathy. Pregabalin is pharmacologically similar to gabapentin, and like gabapentin, it is a structural analog of γ-aminobutyric acid (GABA), although the exact mechanism underlying its analgesic efficacy remains unclear. Both agents are thought to influence glutamate release through alterations of voltage-gated calcium channels (Frampton and Scott 2004). Pregabalin is primarily eliminated by renal excretion; dose modifications are required in patients with impaired renal function.

Carbamazepine is FDA approved for use in trigeminal neuralgia; divalproex sodium and topiramate have both been indicated for migraine prophylaxis. Along with phenytoin, carbamazepine and valproate have been shown to be efficacious in chronic neuropathic pain (Galer 1995; Maciewicz et al. 1985; Swerdlow 1984).

Emerging evidence suggests the potential analgesic roles of newer ACDs (i.e., lamotrigine, oxcarbazepine, tiagabine, topiramate, and zonisamide) (Galer 1995; Khoromi et al. 2005; Novak et al. 2001; Pappagallo 2003), which offer greater tolerability than some of the older ACDs. Although these agents demonstrate some promise with regard to potential utility in neuropathic states (Remillard 1994; Solaro et al. 2001; Zakrzewska et al. 1997), their utility and safety among pain patients require further investigation. These newer agents may offer better tolerability over other ACDs (e.g., carbamazepine) and may be useful for patients with intractable pain or pain that is poorly responsive to other agents.

As with most psychopharmacologic agents, low initial doses of ACDs should be employed and the doses increased gradually while monitoring for any intolerance or adverse events. Pain-mitigating doses are comparable with those employed for anticonvulsant efficacy. Common adverse effects of ACDs are sedation, fatigue, and GI and motor complications. Table 5–10 lists selected ACDs and their common side effects (Leo and Narendran 1999; Swerdlow 1984).

Considering Treatment Options: Antidepressant, Anticonvulsant, or Both?

Because several ACDs have received FDA approval for use in selected pain states, it is perhaps an inclination of many pain practitioners to prescribe an ACD when confronting the pain associated with neuropathy. However, given the efficacy of antidepressants in a number of chronic pain conditions, it is nonetheless important to consider when to use antidepressants and/or ACDs when treating a particular patient. Considerations of medication selection include tolerability of side effects and safety of use of particular medications in the context of the patient's comorbid medical conditions (Leo 2006).

It is often difficult to elicit sufficient funding from pharmaceutical companies to conduct head-to-head comparisons of various agents in pain treatment. One means of bypassing this is to compare analgesic efficacy of different agents across several studies, using the number-needed-to-treat (NNT)

Table 5–10. Side effects of anticonvulsants

Carbamazepine	Valproate
Sedation	Nausea, heartburn, indigestion
Nystagmus, diplopia, ataxia	Vomiting, diarrhea
Nausea, vomiting	Sedation
Myoclonus	Weight gain
Elevated liver enzymes	Tremor
Hyponatremia, SIADH	Rash
Rash	Hair loss
Leukopenia, neutropenia	Thrombocytopenia
Aplastic anemia	Hepatotoxicity
Gabapentin	Pancreatitis
Sedation	Phenytoin
Dizziness, ataxia	Nausea/vomiting
Fatigue	Ataxia
Nystagmus, diplopia	Diplopia
Headache	Hirsutism
Tremor	Gingival hyperplasia
Nausea, vomiting	Confusion
Lamotrigine	
Dizziness	
Ataxia, diplopia, blurred vision	
Sedation	
Headache	
Vomiting	
Rash, Stevens-Johnson syndrome	

Note. SIADH = syndrome of inappropriate antidiuretic hormone.

formula. As shown in the equation in Figure 5–2, the NNT is calculated by considering the proportion of patients who achieve at least 50% relief with the use of an analgesic agent and taking from that value those achieving at least 50% relief with placebo. The difference is then divided into 1. The value of the NNT assigned is an indicator of usefulness, with 1 being ideal and higher numbers reflecting less efficacy. Stated another way, the NNT provides an estimate of the number of patients who need to be given a medication to obtain one patient who achieves at least 50% relief.

The NNT was calculated for antidepressants and anticonvulsants in two meta-analyses of multiple placebo-controlled studies involving patients with neuropathy (Collins et al. 2000; Sindrup and Jensen 1999) (see Table 5–11).

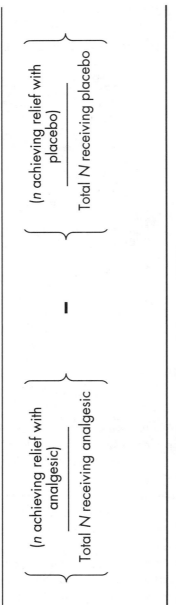

Figure 5–2.   Equation for calculating number-needed-to-treat (NNT).
Source.   McQuay HJ, Moore RA: "Methods of Therapeutic Trials," in *Textbook of Pain*, 4th Edition. Edited by Wall PD, Melzack R. Edinburgh, Churchill Livingstone, 1999, p. 1128.

Table 5–11. Number-needed-to-treat (NNT) values obtained from two meta-analyses assessing antidepressant and anticonvulsant efficacy in neuropathy

| | Collins et al. 2000 | | Sindrup and Jensen 1999 | |
	Medication	NNT	Medication	NNT
Diabetic neuropathy	Anticonvulsants	2.7	TCAs	2.4
	Antidepressants	3.4	Carbamazepine	3.3
			Gabapentin	3.7
			SSRIs	6.7
Postherpetic neuralgia	Antidepressants	2.1	TCAs	2.3
	Anticonvulsants	3.2	Gabapentin	3.2

Note. TCA = tricyclic antidepressant; SSRI = selective serotonin reuptake inhibitor.
Source. Data from Collins SL, Moore RA, McQuay HJ, et al.: "Antidepressants and Anticonvulsants for Diabetic Neuropathy and Postherpetic Neuralgia: A Quantitative Systematic Review." *Journal of Pain Symptom Management* 20:449–458, 2000; Sindrup SH, Jensen TS: "Efficacy of Pharmacological Treatments of Neuropathic Pain: An Update and Effect Related to Mechanism of Drug Action." *Pain* 83:389–400, 1999.

Essentially, for both antidepressants and anticonvulsants, three patients would need to be treated in order for one of them to achieve 50% pain relief. TCAs tended to fare better than SSRIs and, to some extent, anticonvulsants. However, adverse effects were more common with antidepressant use, particularly TCAs, than with anticonvulsant use (Collins et al. 2000).

Selection of an antidepressant might be based on the fact that several of these agents have direct pain-mitigating effects, independent of effects on mood. However, for the patient with comorbid depression and/or anxiety that may accompany and exacerbate pain, selection of an antidepressant might be most promising to address pain and mood disturbances simultaneously. In addition, antidepressants might be a consideration when there is a desire to simultaneously address sleep and appetite disturbances accompanying painful conditions.

ACDs have mood-stabilizing effects and are useful for pain patients with psychiatric comorbidities, such as bipolar disorder, schizoaffective disorder, and impulsivity arising from dementia (Leo and Narendran 1999). Thus, patients with mood disturbances, impulsivity, and unpredictable aggression along with coexistent chronic pain may be ideal candidates for ACD selection.

Because of the differences in the pain-relieving effects of ACDs as compared with antidepressants, it is plausible that ACDs would be workable alternatives for patients with persisting pain despite optimal antidepressant use or patients for whom antidepressant use has proved intolerable. Alternatively, simultaneous administration of antidepressants and ACDs could be used, because the analgesic mechanisms of these classes of agents complement each other. When antidepressants and ACDs are coadministered, lower doses of the antidepressant, the ACD, or both are possible, perhaps allowing analgesia to occur while circumventing the higher doses of either agent that predispose a person to adverse effects.

The presence of certain comorbidities may preclude the use of an antidepressant or ACD. Heart block, arrhythmias, and severe cardiac disease prohibit use of TCAs. In the event of renal dysfunction, doses of venlafaxine, carbamazepine, oxcarbazepine, gabapentin, pregabalin, and topiramate would need to be reduced, and if the renal dysfunction is severe enough, use of these agents may be precluded. For patients with hepatic disease, doses of carbamazepine, oxcarbazepine, and lamotrigine should be reduced. TCAs may conceivably exacerbate encephalopathy associated with hepatic disease.

Antihistamines

Histamines have been implicated in a number of pain states (e.g., headache and inflammatory pains) because of their role in facilitating inflammatory processes (e.g., prostaglandin production). Antihistamine effects, therefore, could be expected to reduce pain mediated by inflammatory processes. Furthermore, antihistamine effects appear to augment opiate receptor binding of opioid analgesics (Rumore and Schlichting 1986). Thus, antihistamines might be seen both as augmenting agents to further the effects of other analgesics (e.g., opiates) and as solitary agents on their own. Used alone, antihistamines such as diphenhydramine and hydroxyzine appear to have a ceiling effect. Additionally, these agents may be particularly useful in patients, given their sedative, antiemetic, and anxiolytic properties. Antihistamines are fairly well tolerated, with few respiratory or GI side effects. These agents may be sedating, however, and may intensify appetite; therefore, they may be problematic in patients for whom excess weight might exacerbate current pain disorders (e.g., obese patients with low back pain) and in those with musculoskeletal pains for whom weight loss might reduce discomfort and deconditioning. An additional concern is that confusion and delirium may arise from use of antihistamines. Antihistamines may need to be initiated at low doses, with dose increases as tolerated and warranted to address pain, sleep, and so forth. For example, hydroxyzine may be initiated at a dosage of 25 mg/day, and the dosage may be increased slowly as tolerated.

Benzodiazepines and Anxiolytics

Benzodiazepines have been employed acutely to mitigate pain arising from muscle spasm (e.g., after spinal cord injury). The presumption is that patients with marked anxiety are prone to heightened muscle tension, which may exacerbate musculoskeletal pain. Other uses for benzodiazepines have included treatment of restless legs syndrome, tension headache, and neuropathy (Bartusch et al. 1996; Bouckoms and Litman 1985; Dellemijn and Fields 1994). Clonazepam, a long-acting benzodiazepine, might be effective in patients with neuropathic pain in which allodynia (painful sensations elicited by normally nonnoxious stimuli, such as a bedsheet pulled up along the legs) appears to be a prominent feature (Bouckoms and Litman 1985).

Protracted benzodiazepine use among patients with chronic pain is controversial in that benzodiazepines are GABA agonists and as such may influence 5-HT neurotransmitter release, attenuating opioid analgesia (Nemmani and Mogil 2003), with the potential for increasing pain sensitivity. In addition, protracted benzodiazepine use may be counterproductive. In a study of patients with chronic pain referred to a tertiary pain center, regression analysis revealed that long-term benzodiazepine use predicted low activity levels, high utilization of ambulatory medical services, and high disability levels (Ciccone et al. 2000). Use of benzodiazepines must be undertaken cautiously, because these agents may contribute to excessive sedation, gait instability, and memory impairments (Fishbain et al. 1992; King and Strain 1990).

Buspirone is an anxiolytic agent that differs from benzodiazepines, mediating an antianxiety effect through the $5-HT_{1A}$ receptor. One study reported that patients with neuropathic pain tended not to respond favorably to buspirone treatment (Kishore-Kumar et al. 1989). However, in patients with severe anxiety that may aggravate pain experiences, a trial of buspirone to mitigate anxiety may be warranted.

Table 5–12.   Triptans available for abortive migraine treatment

Duration of effect	Agent	Formulation(s)	Dosing
Long acting	Eletriptan	Oral	20–40 mg[a]
	Frovatriptan	Oral	2.5 mg[b]
	Naratriptan	Oral	1–2.5 mg[c]
Short acting	Almotriptan	Oral	6.25–12.5 mg[a]
	Rizatriptan	Oral	5–10 mg[a]
		Rapid dissolving	5–10 mg[a]
	Sumatriptan	Oral	25–50 mg[a]
		Nasal spray	5–20 mg[a]
		Subcutaneous injection	6 mg[d]
	Zolmitriptan	Oral	2.5–5 mg[a]
		Nasal spray	5 mg[a]
		Rapid dissolving	2.5–5 mg[a]

Note.   Generally no more than two doses should be employed in 24 hours, and no more often than 2 days per week.
[a]May repeat after 2 hours.
[b]May repeat after 6–8 hours.
[c]May repeat after 4 hours.
[d]May repeat after 1 hour.

Triptans

The triptans are 5-$HT_{1B/1D}$ receptor agonists used for acute migraine treatment (see Table 5–12). The triptans are effective in aborting migraine through influences on cranial vasoconstriction, peripheral neural inhibition, and inhibition of trigeminocervical (second-order) neurons. Ideally, these agents should be employed early in the onset of migraine for greatest effect (Goadsby et al. 2002).

The side effects of triptans may include paresthesias, dizziness, flushing, neck stiffness, and warm sensations extending over the head, neck, and chest. Angina, chest pain and pressure, and myocardial ischemia are possible because of the triptans' potential for coronary vasoconstriction. Triptans should be avoided in patients with uncontrolled hypertension, coronary artery disease, Prinzmetal's angina, cerebrovascular disorders, or peripheral vascular disease (Goadsby et al. 2002; Matchar et al. 2002).

Sumatriptan and other triptans may be taken concurrently with serotonergic antidepressants; however, there have been a few case reports of serotonin syndrome arising from such combinations (Mathew et al. 1996; Putnam et al. 1999). Use of MAOIs may impede the metabolism of sumatriptan and rizatriptan (McEvoy 2006).

Stimulants

Stimulants may have analgesic effects when combined with opioids (Forrest et al. 1977; Laska et al. 1984). Dextroamphetamine (5–15 mg two or three times daily) or methylphenidate (5–15 mg two to four times daily) has been used to augment opiate analgesia. These drugs have also been used to reduce the sedation, dysphoria, and cognitive inefficiency that may accompany opiate use. Both pemoline (up to 75 mg/day) and caffeine (65 mg two or three times daily) have likewise been used for such purposes. However, use of stimulants may be limited by intervening adverse effects, including overstimulation (e.g., anxiety, insomnia, paranoia), appetite suppression (problematic in patients who are undernourished and cachectic), and confusion. Additionally, in persons who are predisposed to motor abnormalities, tics and other dyskinetic movements may be exacerbated. When these drugs are taken in overdose, an extreme form of these adverse effects may occur, resulting potentially in hypertension, arrhythmias, seizures, hallucinations (including formication), delirium, and death. Contraindications for stimulant use include glaucoma, poorly controlled hypertension, arrhythmias and cardiovascular disorders, anorexia, seizure disorders, and hyperthyroidism. Pemoline has been removed from the market at the urging of the FDA because of concerns about liver dysfunction and hepatotoxicity associated with its use.

The use of stimulants has been limited because of fears regarding abuse and addiction. Caution is advised in patients with current or preexisting substance use disorders, especially prior stimulant abuse (e.g., cocaine). Both dextroamphetamine and methylphenidate are Schedule II medications under federal regulatory control. Physicians may be reluctant to make use of these agents because they fear possible misinterpretation by government agencies and punitive measures that may be taken when these agents are prescribed.

Modafinil recently has been studied for its utility in addressing opioid-induced sedation and postoperative fatigue related to general anesthesia use

(Larijani et al. 2004; Reissig and Rybarczyk 2005). Generally, 200–400 mg daily may be required for such purposes. Lower doses (e.g., 100 mg daily) are recommended in patients with hepatic impairments. Adverse effects are similar to those associated with other sympathomimetic agents.

Neuroleptics

There have been a limited number of studies demonstrating the efficacy of various neuroleptics (e.g., fluphenazine) in chronic pain states. These agents have been found to be useful in certain cases of neuropathic pain (Gomez-Perez et al. 1985). In animal models, clozapine and risperidone were found to have analgesic effects, but olanzapine had only a modest antinociceptive influence (Schreiber et al. 1997, 1999). In two small clinical case series, olanzapine was effective in reducing the severity ratings of recurrent migrane and tension headache refractory to other interventions (Silberstein et al. 2000) and cancer pain (Fishbain et al. 2004). In another small series, olanzapine was useful in mitigating cancer pain and reducing opiate requirements among these patients (Khojainova et al. 2002). One antipsychotic, methotrimeprazine, has demonstrated analgesic activity comparable to low-dose morphine (Beaver et al. 1966). Methotrimeprazine is available in Canada and Europe but not in the United States. It appears that the limited data on the efficacy of neuroleptics, the abundance of other agents to choose from, and the side effects of the neuroleptics would warrant avoiding these agents. The risks of neuroleptic use (e.g., extrapyramidal side effects, tardive dyskinesia) appear to far outweigh any analgesic efficacy. Use of neuroleptics should probably be confined to the patient who has delirium and psychosis, although the potential role of atypical antipsychotics in refractory conditions may warrant further investigation (Fishbain et al. 2004).

Mexiletine

Mexiletine is one of many antiarrhythmics that may be used for pain; it has the advantage of being administered orally. The risk is that patients may experience untoward cardiac effects (i.e., the drug may influence cardiac rhythms). Patients with heart block may be particularly vulnerable to adverse cardiac effects brought on by mexiletine. Mexiletine has been used to treat neuropathic pain. The medication is initiated at a dosage of 150 mg/day given in divided doses, and the dosage is increased gradually (approximately every 3–7 days) to a maximum of 1,200 mg/day, given in divided doses.

Alpha$_2$-Adrenergic Agonists

α_2-Adrenergic agonists (e.g., clonidine) are available for epidural administration for neuropathic pain (Eisenach et al. 1995). Hypotension and bradycardia may result from use of these agents, but the risk is reduced if low doses are used. Adverse effects include hemodynamic instability. There is a risk of rebound hypertension with acute withdrawal of therapy. Topical clonidine gel is being developed for use in neuropathic pain states. Tizanidine, another α_2-adrenergic agonist, is used for muscle relaxation.

N-Methyl-D-Aspartate Antagonists

Although the mechanisms are complex and have yet to be fully elucidated, research implicates the excitatory neurotransmitter glutamate in the development and maintenance of chronic pain. Some evidence suggests that NMDA antagonists (i.e., dextromethorphan, ketamine, memantine, and amantadine) may therefore have a role in mitigating chronic pain, including neuropathy, chronic phantom pain, and fibromyalgia, and pain associated with spinal cord injury (Fisher et al. 2000; Sang et al. 2002). However, the analgesic effects in various trials have been inconsistent (Eisenberg et al. 1998; Enarson et al. 1999).

The side effects associated with the NMDA antagonists include sedation, dry mouth, headache, and constipation; in some cases these effects may be prohibitively severe, limiting usefulness (e.g., ketamine may produce dissociation, hallucinations, frightening nightmares, and delirium) (Eide et al. 1994). Ketamine at a dosage of 50–60 mg four to six times daily (taken in juice or oral suspension) may produce pain relief without incurring these serious effects. Ketamine's hallucinogenic properties have rendered it popular with drug abusers (Dillon et al. 2003). Long-term use of ketamine is not currently advocated, partly because the long-term effects are unknown. It may result in long-term cognitive changes, hepatic dysfunction, and gastric ulcers.

Widely available as an over-the-counter medication, dextromethorphan is notable for its cough-suppressing effects. It is a low-affinity NMDA receptor antagonist that, when combined with opiate analgesics, may enhance opiate analgesia and reduce opiate tolerance (Elliott et al. 1994). Analgesic effects require dosing at rates substantially higher than those for antitussive effects. Dextromethorphan augments 5-HT in the CNS. Consequently, combination with serotonergic antidepressants (e.g., SSRIs) may predispose a patient to serotonin syndrome.

At a dosage of 200–300 mg orally per day, amantadine may have several untoward effects associated with other NMDA antagonists (e.g., nervousness, depression, concentration disturbances, sleep disturbances). Memantine may be better tolerated than other NMDA antagonists and, given its utility among patients with dementia, may be particularly ideal in patients with dementia and complicating pain conditions.

Methadone, too, has NMDA antagonist properties. One isomer of methadone acts by blocking NMDA receptors (Shimoyama et al. 1997), which may contribute to the fact that methadone maintains analgesic efficacy as compared with other opioids and, therefore, might not require opiate rotations (Gorman et al. 1997; see sections "Agents With Multiple Uses" and "Tolerance, Dependence, and Pseudoaddiction" in this chapter).

Corticosteroids

Corticosteroids have been used in pain states associated with chronic medical conditions (e.g., inflammatory pain, irritable bowel, spinal cord compression, headache caused by increased intracranial pressure). The corticosteroids have also been used to treat cancer-related pain, especially in patients who have bone metastases, hepatic or biliary involvement from tumor, or epidural metastases with spinal cord compression. Side effects associated with corticosteroid use are summarized in Table 5–13. The benefits of steroid use must be weighed against the risks associated with long-term use. When administered intramuscularly, intrathecally, or epidurally, corticosteroids may be used at substantially lower doses than when administered orally. The lower doses may help to reduce potential systemic adverse effects.

Corticosteroids inhibit the release of phospholipase A, necessary for the conversion of arachidonic acid to leukotrienes and prostaglandins. The latter

Table 5–13. Side effects of corticosteroid use in pain

Immune suppression (increased infection risk, *Candida* infection)

Myopathy

Sodium imbalance–electrolyte disturbance

Fluid overload (congestive heart failure, peripheral edema, pulmonary edema)

Glucose intolerance (iatrogenic diabetes, worsening of preexisting diabetes mellitus)

Gastrointestinal disturbances (bleeding, peritonitis)

Skin breakdown

Neuropsychiatric disturbances (mood, perceptual, and cognitive disturbances)

are responsible for inflammatory pains; they also produce reduced ectopic firing of neurons (e.g., after amputation), producing phantom limb pain. Corticosteroids inhibit activity of C fibers but not of other sensory fibers (e.g., Aβ fibers). Each of the corticosteroids produces equivalent analgesia (Bruera et al. 1985; Ettinger and Portenoy 1988). Selection of one corticosteroid over another may be based on the tolerability and the desire to avoid serious mineralocorticoid effects (e.g., such as those seen with dexamethasone). Patients in whom steroid use might be contraindicated include those with severe cardiac compromise, a predisposition to congestive heart failure, severe osteoporosis, diabetes mellitus, or electrolyte disturbances.

Muscle Antispasmodics

Muscle antispasmodics include true muscle relaxants (e.g., baclofen, dantrolene) along with agents in which the mechanism of action is unclear (e.g., carisoprodol, cyclobenzaprine, methocarbamol, orphenadrine). Some of these agents may suppress polysynaptic reflexes and thereby reduce pain, but they do not influence skeletal muscles per se.

Generally, antispasmodic agents are to be used for acute pain arising from muscle strain or injury (see Table 5–14). Baclofen might be indicated for more chronic pain arising from muscle spasticity (e.g., after stroke or severe spinal cord injury). The utility of these agents for long-term use is unclear. There may be abuse potential associated with carisoprodol and methocarbamol. Carisoprodol is metabolized to meprobamate; therefore, ongoing use might possibly lead to meprobamate dependence. Abrupt discontinuation of carisoprodol may produce mild withdrawal, including abdominal cramps, insomnia, nausea,

Table 5–14.   Dosing of muscle relaxants

Agent	Dosage recommendation
Baclofen	5 mg tid, up to 40–80 mg/day
Carisoprodol	350 mg qid
Chlorzoxazone	250–750 mg tid to qid
Cyclobenzaprine	10 mg tid, up to a maximum of 60 mg/day
Orphenadrine	100 mg bid
Methocarbamol	1,500 mg qid for 72 hours, then 1,000 mg qid
Diazepam	2–10 mg tid to qid
Tizanidine	2–8 mg tid to qid

headache, and anxiety. Carisoprodol is contraindicated in patients with acute intermittent porphyria. Severe psychiatric disturbances, such as psychotic depression, have been reported in association with baclofen use (Sommer and Petrides 1992); delirium may result from its abrupt discontinuation (Leo and Baer 2005).

Side effects often associated with muscle antispasmodics include somnolence and anticholinergic effects. Patients should be advised that such agents may impede their ability to operate heavy machinery or to drive a vehicle. Combination with other sedative agents (i.e., alcohol, sedative-hypnotics, benzodiazepines, barbiturates) may produce additive sedative effects. Chlorzoxazone has been associated with hepatotoxicity and might therefore be an unwise selection as a muscle relaxant for long-term use. This risk may be increased if the drug is combined with other agents with hepatotoxic effects (e.g., acetaminophen or nefazodone).

Baclofen is an agonist of $GABA_B$ receptors. It may also suppress the release of excitatory amino acids such as glutamate and inhibit substance P. Baclofen has been used primarily for spasticity, but it also may be helpful in reducing neuropathic pains (e.g., of trigeminal neuralgia) and other neuropathies. The routes of administration are oral and intrathecal.

Tizanidine is an α_2-adrenergic agonist (like clonidine) that may function to reduce muscle spasticity by decreasing the spinal excitatory amino acid release, which may have an impact on muscle contractility.

Cyclobenzaprine is used in treating fibromyalgia. It has a tricyclic chemical structure and is accompanied by anticholinergic side effects. Cyclobenzaprine is contraindicated in persons with ischemic heart disease, congestive heart failure, cardiac arrhythmias, or heart block. It is extremely lethal in overdose, and caution must be undertaken when prescribing this agent to persons with risk factors for suicide. Cyclobenzaprine must never be used in conjunction with MAOIs because of risks of toxic reactions, which include hyperthermia.

Topical Agents

Topical agents allow for pain relief through direct application of analgesics to the skin, presumably at the direct source of pain, thereby bypassing significant systemic effects.

Capsaicin

Derived from red chili peppers, capsaicin has efficacy in reducing arthritic pain and some neuropathic pain states. The mechanism for pain relief is thought to be derived from depletion of substance P at sites of pain. Alternatively, counterirritation mechanisms (see Chapter 2, "Sensory Pathways of Pain and Acute Versus Chronic Pain," of this book) may be involved. Some patients find the burning sensations at the site of application to be too uncomfortable, precluding use.

Lidocaine Patch

The lidocaine patch functions to ameliorate pain when the patch is applied to intact skin surfaces affected by pain related to neuropathy or myofascial or osteoarthritis-related pain. The local anesthetic is thought to mitigate pain by influencing voltage-sensitive sodium channels to stabilize neural membranes. The patch provides approximately 12 hours of relief, requiring reapplication of additional patches for refractory and recurrent pain. The patch is generally well tolerated, but irritation and erythema may occur at the site of application.

Eutectic Mixture of Local Anesthetics

A eutectic mixture of local anesthetics (EMLA) is a solution consisting of two local anesthetics (lidocaine and prilocaine). This topically applied anesthetic agent has marked analgesic properties (Kapelushnik et al. 1990). It is customarily employed in conditions involving skin surgery, such as curettage of skin lesions, split-thickness graft harvesting, collagen implants, removal of warts and port-wine stains, and so forth. Application of EMLA may cause localized vasoconstriction of skin. In addition, methemoglobinemia and hypoxia may also arise as a response to prilocaine contained in the EMLA solution. Edema and erythema may develop as well, particularly when EMLA is applied to diseased tissues or skin.

Herbal Agents

Use of herbal agents has become increasingly popular in the treatment of pain (Kaufman et al. 2002); agents used for a variety of pain complaints are listed in Table 5–15. Often framed as "natural remedies," herbal agents are often believed to be safe and devoid of adverse effects and therefore may go unreported. It is important to make inquiries into the patient's use of herbs, because these may be associated with significant adverse effects and drug interactions when unknowingly combined with prescribed medications (Ernst 2000).

Cannabinoids

Animal models suggest that cannabinoids have potent antinociceptive effects (Fox et al. 2001). Analgesic effects are thought to be mediated by binding to cannabinoid receptors within the CNS (CB1 receptor) and in the periphery (CB2 receptor). Additionally, cannabinoids are also capable of influencing serotonergic and dopaminergic activity and endogenous opiates, thereby influencing pain transmission. Cannabinoids have been advocated for use in migraine prophylaxis and neuropathy and for anti-inflammatory purposes. For example, dronabinol (10 mg/day) was effective in reducing spontaneous pain associated with multiple sclerosis and was more effective than placebo in a small study (Svendsen et al. 2004). Side effects were common, unfortunately, and included fatigue, dizziness, headache, muscle ache, and potential mood disturbances (e.g., anxiety, mania). Several oral cannabinoids are currently under development for anti-inflammatory and neuropathic pain conditions; development of agents with specificity for the peripheral CB2 receptor may provide sufficient analgesia while avoiding untoward effects associated with central (CB1) receptor activity (e.g., fatigue, dizziness).

Table 5–15.   Herbal agents used for pain

Herb	Use	Comment
Black cohash	Menstrual pain	Can produce adverse gastrointestinal (GI) effects; and abdominal, headache, and joint pain; can increase intensity of contraceptives
Chamomile	Anti-inflammatory	Acts as emetic; may interfere with anticoagulants
Evening primrose oil	Anti-inflammatory; rheumatoid arthritis, migraine	May trigger temporal lobe epilepsy; unsafe in patients taking phenothiazine antipsychotics
Feverfew	Anti-inflammatory; migraine	Interacts with antithrombotic agents
Ginkgo biloba	Claudication-related pain	Can produce GI distress, headache
Goldenseal	Anti-inflammatory	Can produce seizure, B vitamin deficiencies; induces abortion in pregnancy
Kava	Antispasmodic	Can potentiate sedation from barbiturates and alcohol
Topical St. John's wort	Anti-inflammatory	GI distress; can produce serotonin syndrome if combined with selective serotonin reuptake inhibitors (uncertain if this is a risk with topical applications)
Valerian	Migraine headache	GI distress, insomnia; interferes with anticonvulsants and anxiolytics

Placebo Effects

The physiologic aspects of pain are inextricably linked with cognitive and emotional aspects. Thus, it is not uncommon to find that many patients with pain may derive relief from placebos (i.e., agents or interventions believed to be inefficacious). In experimental paradigms, placebo effects of pain relief were encountered in 15%–58% of patients (Turner et al. 1994). Factors mediating the placebo effect include patient expectations and hopes for relief. Placebo effects are expected to be enhanced by the conviction of the clinician of the expected relief as well as the costs of the intervention. It is possible that administration of a placebo may reduce patient anxiety and distress, thereby mitigating pain awareness. On the other hand, placebo administration has at times been associated with increases in endogenous opiate release within the CNS, thereby mitigating pain.

Caution is advised not to ascribe any influence to a treatment that is nothing more than the natural course and variability intrinsic to a disease state. Thus, experimental approaches assessing the efficacy of a treatment will naturally require a placebo arm and perhaps a wait-list control group to tease out those changes that occur over time. In addition, the clinician is cautioned about dismissing the complaints of a patient who appears to respond positively to a placebo. The positive response does not inherently imply that the allegations of pain are psychologically based.

Key Points

- Opiates have been the mainstay of treatment of acute and terminal pain states. Use in chronic, nonmalignant pain states may be indicated, but for many clinicians, such use raises concerns regarding dependence.
- Factors influencing choice of an opiate analgesic include pain severity, side-effect profiles, the possibilities of drug interactions, and concerns related to use of opiates in patients with medical comorbidities.
- Analgesic agents employed in mild pain include acetaminophen, NSAIDs, and celecoxib. Safety of the use of such agents must be considered before they are employed for the long term.

- Adjuvant analgesic agents employed for chronic pain include several psychoactive agents, such as antidepressants, anticonvulsants, antihistamines, benzodiazepines, stimulants, and, in selected refractory cases, neuroleptics.
- Antidepressants have direct pain-mitigating effects apart from influences on mood. Among the antidepressants, those with simultaneous NE and 5-HT influences appear to have greater analgesic utility as compared with agents with primarily single-neurotransmitter influences. Antidepressants can produce analgesia faster and at doses far lower than those required for antidepressant effects. The pain-mitigating effects of antidepressants remain a subject of intensive investigation and are thought to involve a number of supraspinal, spinal, and peripheral processes.
- On the basis of two meta-analyses of multiple placebo-controlled studies involving patients with neuropathy, the number-needed-to-treat calculations derived for antidepressants and anticonvulsants are comparable; however, adverse effects were more common with antidepressants, particularly TCAs, than with anticonvulsants. Selection of an antidepressant versus an anticonvulsant might theoretically be based on the presence of mood disorders and other psychiatric comorbidities accompanying pain amenable to medications of a particular class, the potential for drug interactions, and the presence of medical conditions that may contraindicate use of agents of a particular class.
- Several analgesic agents have been associated with potential for psychiatric sequelae—for example, opiates and benzodiazepines (depression, delirium, cognitive impairments, withdrawal after sudden cessation), NSAIDs (depression), tramadol (delirium secondary to seizures), stimulants (anxiety, decreased appetite), ketamine and dextromethorphan (hallucinations, psychosis), triptans (serotonin syndrome if combined with serotonergic antidepressants), baclofen (delirium secondary to abrupt withdrawal), and cannabinoids (anxiety, mania).
- Herbal agents have become increasingly popular in treating a variety of pain complaints; however, caution is advised because of concerns over adverse effects and potential drug interactions when herbs are combined with prescribed medications.
- Analgesic agents with abuse or addiction potential or diversion appeal include opiates, benzodiazepines, tramadol, stimulants, selected NMDA antagonists, and selected muscle relaxants.

References

Abbott FV, Hong Y, Blier P: Persisting sensitization of the behavioural response to formalin-induced injury through activation of serotonin$_{2A}$ receptors. Neuroscience 77:575–584, 1997

Abernethy DR, Greenblatt DJ, Steel K, et al: Impairment of hepatic drug oxidation by propoxyphene. Ann Intern Med 97:223–224, 1982

Ansari A: The efficacy of newer antidepressants in the treatment of chronic pain: a review of current literature. Harv Rev Psychiatry 7:257–277, 2000

Arnold LM, Lu Y, Crofford LJ, et al: A double-blind, multicenter trial comparing duloxetine with placebo in the treatment of fibromyalgia patients with or without major depressive disorder. Arthritis Rheum 50:2974–2984, 2004

Baba H, Shimoji K, Yoshimura M: Norepinephrine facilitates inhibitory transmission in substantia gelatinosa of adult rat spinal cord (part 1): effects on axon terminals of GABAergic and glycinergic neurons. Anesthesiology 92:473–484, 2000

Bartusch SL, Sanders BJ, D'Alessio JG, et al: Clonazepam for the treatment of lancinating phantom limb pain. Clin J Pain 12:59–62, 1996

Beaver WT, Wallenstein SL, Houde RW, et al: A comparison of the analgesic effects of methotrimeprazine and morphine in patients with cancer. Clin Pharmacol Ther 7:436–466, 1966

Bendtsen L, Jensen R: Mirtazapine is effective in the prophylactic treatment of chronic tension-type headache. Neurology 62:1706–1711, 2004

Bouckoms A: Psychiatric aspects of pain in the critically ill, in Problems in Critical Care. Edited by Wise MG. Philadelphia, PA, JB Lippincott, 1988

Bouckoms AJ, Litman RE: Clonazepam in the treatment of neuralgic pain syndrome. Psychosomatics 26:933–936, 1985

Browning CH: Nonsteroidal anti-inflammatory drugs and severe psychiatric side effects. Int J Psychiatry Med 26:25–34, 1996

Bruera E, Roca E, Cedaro L, et al: Action of oral methylprednisolone in terminal cancer patients: a prospective randomized double-blind study. Cancer Treat Rep 69:751–754, 1985

Buckley FP, Sizemore WA, Charlton JE: Medication management in patients with chronic nonmalignant pain: a review of the use of a drug withdrawal protocol. Pain 26:153–165, 1986

Cassem NH: Pain (Current Topics in Medicine, Vol. 2), in Scientific American Medicine. Edited by Rubenstein E, Federman DD. New York, Scientific American, 1989

Ciccone DS, Just N, Bandilla EB, et al: Psychological correlates of opioid use in patients with chronic nonmalignant pain: a preliminary test of the downhill spiral hypothesis. J Pain Symptom Manage 20:180–192, 2000

Collins SL, Moore RA, McQuay HJ, et al: Antidepressants and anticonvulsants for diabetic neuropathy and postherpetic neuralgia: a quantitative systematic review. J Pain Symptom Manage 20:449–458, 2000

Dellemijn PL, Fields HL: Do benzodiazepines have a role in chronic pain management? Pain 57:137–152, 1994

Diamond S, Freitag FG: The use of fluoxetine in the treatment of headache. Clin J Pain 5:200–201, 1989

Dillon P, Copeland J, Jansen K: Patterns of use and harms associated with non-medical ketamine use. Drug Alcohol Depend 69:23–28, 2003

Eide PK, Jorum E, Stubhaug A, et al: Relief of post-herpetic neuralgia with the N-methyl-aspartic acid receptor antagonist ketamine: a double-blind cross-over comparison with morphine and placebo. Pain 58:347–354, 1994

Eisenach JC, DuPen SL, Dubois M, et al: Epidural clonidine analgesia for intractable cancer pain. Pain 61:391–399, 1995

Eisenberg E, Kleiser A, Dotort A, et al: The NMDA (N-methyl-D-aspartate) receptor antagonist memantine in the treatment of postherpetic neuralgia: a double-blind, placebo-controlled study. Eur J Pain 2:321–327, 1998

Elliott K, Hynansky A, Inturrisi CE: Dextromethorphan attenuates and reverses analgesic tolerance to morphine. Pain 59:361–368, 1994

Enarson MC, Hays H, Woodroffe MA: Clinical experience with oral ketamine. J Pain Symptom Manage 17:384–386, 1999

Ernst E: Herb–drug interactions: potentially important but woefully under-researched. Eur J Clin Pharmacol 56:523–524, 2000

Ettinger AB, Portenoy RK: The use of corticosteroids in the treatment of symptoms associated with cancer. J Pain Symptom Manage 3:99–103, 1988

Fields HL, Basbaum AI: Central nervous system mechanisms of pain modulation, in Textbook of Pain, 4th Edition. Edited by Wall PD, Melzack R. Edinburgh, Scotland, Churchill Livingstone, 1999, pp 309–329

Finlayson RE, Maruta T, Morse RM, et al: Substance dependence and chronic pain: profile of 50 patients treated in an alcohol and drug dependence unit. Pain 26:167–174, 1986

Fishbain DA, Rosomoff HL, Rosomoff RS: Detoxification of nonopiate drugs in the chronic pain setting and clonidine opiate detoxification. Clin J Pain 8:191–203, 1992

Fishbain DA, Cutler RB, Lewis J, et al: Do the second-generation "atypical neuroleptics" have analgesic properties? A structured evidence-based review. Pain Med 5:359–365, 2004

Fisher K, Coderre TJ, Hagen NA: Targeting the N-methyl-D-aspartate receptor for chronic pain management: preclinical animal studies, recent clinical experience and future research directions. J Pain Symptom Manage 20:358–373, 2000

Forrest WH, Brown BW, Brown CR, et al: Dextroamphetamine with morphine for the treatment of postoperative pain. N Engl J Med 296:712–715, 1977

Fox A, Kesingland A, Gentry C, et al: The role of central and peripheral cannabinoid$_1$ receptors in the antihyperalgesic activity of cannabinoids in a model of neuropathic pain. Pain 92:91–100, 2001

Frampton JE, Scott LJ: Pregabalin in the treatment of painful diabetic neuropathy. Drugs 64:2813–2820, 2004

Galer BS: Neuropathic pain of peripheral origin: advances in pharmacologic treatment. Neurology 45 (suppl 9):17–25, 1995

Gerner P, Mujtaba M, Sinnott CJ, et al: Amitriptyline versus bupivacaine in rat sciatic nerve blockade. Anesthesiology 94:661–667, 2001

Goadsby PJ, Lipton RB, Ferrari MD: Drug therapy: migraine—current understanding and treatment. N Engl J Med 346:257–270, 2002

Goldstein DJ, Lu Y, Detke MJ, et al: Duloxetine vs. placebo in patients with painful diabetic neuropathy. Pain 116:109–118, 2005

Gomez-Perez FJ, Rull JA, Dies H, et al: Nortriptyline and fluphenazine in the symptomatic treatment of diabetic neuropathy: a double-blind cross-over study. Pain 23:395–400, 1985

Goodnick PJ, Breakstone K, Khumar A, et al: Nefazodone in diabetic neuropathy: response and biology. Psychosom Med 62:599–600, 2000

Gorman AL, Elliott KJ, Inturrisi CE: The d- and l-isomers of methadone bind to the noncompetitive site on the N-methyl-D-aspartate (NMDA) receptor in rat forebrain and spinal cord. Neurosci Lett 223:5–8, 1997

Gratz SS, Simpson GM: MAOI–narcotic interactions (letter). J Clin Psychiatry 54:439, 1993

Inturrisi CE: Role of opioid analgesics. Am J Med 77(suppl):27–37, 1984

Jaffe JH, Martin WR: Opioid analgesics and antagonists, in The Pharmacological Basis of Therapeutics. Edited by Gilman AG, Rall TW, Nies AS, et al. New York, Pergamon, 1990

Jiang HK, Chang DM: Non-steroidal anti-inflammatory drugs with adverse psychiatric reactions: five case reports. Clin Rheumatol 18:339–345, 1999

Kapelushnik J, Koren G, Solh H, et al: Evaluating the efficacy of EMLA in alleviating pain associated with lumbar puncture; comparison of open and double-blinded protocols in children. Pain 42:31–34, 1990

Kaufman DW, Kelly JP, Rosenberg L, et al: Recent patterns of medication use in the ambulatory adult population of the United States—the Slone Survey. JAMA 287:337–344, 2002

Kawasaki Y, Kumamoto E, Furue H, et al: α2 adrenoceptor-mediated presynaptic inhibition of primary afferent glutamatergic transmission in rat substantia gelatinosa neurons. Anesthesiology 98:682–689, 2003

Keeri-Szanto M: The mode of action of promethazine in potentiating narcotic drugs. Br J Anaesth 46:918–924, 1974

Khojainova N, Santiago-Palma J, Kornick C, et al: Olanzapine in the management of cancer pain. J Pain Symptom Manage 23:346–350, 2002

Khoromi S, Patsalides A, Parada S, et al: Topiramate in chronic lumbar radicular pain. J Pain 6:829–836, 2005

Khurana RC: Treatment of painful diabetic neuropathy with trazodone (letter). JAMA 250:1392, 1983

King SA, Strain J: Benzodiazepine use by chronic pain patients. Clin J Pain 6:143–147, 1990

Kishore-Kumar R, Schafer SC, Lawlor BA, et al: Single doses of the serotonin agonists buspirone and m-chlorophenylpiperazine do not relieve neuropathic pain. Pain 37:223–227, 1989

Krell HV, Leuchter AF, Cook IA, et al: Evaluation of reboxetine, a noradrenergic anti-depressant, for the treatment of fibromyalgia and chronic low back pain. Psychosomatics 46:379–384, 2005

Larijani GE, Goldberg ME, Hojat M, et al: Modafinil improves recovery after general anesthesia. Anesth Analg 98:976–981, 2004

Larson AA, Takemori AE: Effect of fluoxetine hydrochloride (Lilly 110140), a specific inhibitor of serotonin uptake, on morphine analgesia and the development of tolerance. Life Sci 21:1807–1812, 1977

Laska EM, Sunshine A, Mueller F, et al: Caffeine as an analgesic adjuvant. JAMA 251:1711–1718, 1984

Lee RL, Spencer PSJ: Effect of tricyclic antidepressants on analgesic activity in laboratory animals. Postgrad Med J 56 (suppl 1):19–24, 1980

Leo RJ: Treatment considerations in neuropathic pain. Curr Treat Options Neurol 8:389–400, 2006

Leo RJ: Pain disorders, in The American Psychiatric Publishing Textbook of Clinical Psychiatry, 5th Edition. Edited by Hales RE, Yudofsky SC, Gabbard GO. Washington, DC, American Psychiatric Publishing, 2008

Leo RJ, Baer D: Delirium associated with baclofen withdrawal: a review of common presentations and management strategies. Psychosomatics 46:503–507, 2005

Leo RJ, Brooks VL: Clinical potential of milnacipran, a serotonin and norepinephrine reuptake inhibitor, in pain. Curr Opin Investig Drugs 7:637–642, 2006

Leo RJ, Narendran R: Anticonvulsant use in the treatment of bipolar disorder: a primer for primary care physicians. Prim Care Companion J Clin Psychiatry 1:74–84, 1999

Leo RJ, Narendran R, DeGuiseppe B: Methadone detoxification of tramadol dependence. J Subst Abuse Treat 19:297–299, 2000

Maciewicz R, Bouckoms A, Martin JB: Drug therapy of neuropathic pain. Clin J Pain 1:39–49, 1985

Maltbie AA, Cavenar JO, Sullivan JL, et al: Analgesia and haloperidol: a hypothesis. J Clin Psychiatry 40:323–326, 1979

Massie MJ (ed): Pain: What Psychiatrists Need to Know (Review of Psychiatry Series, Vol 19; Oldham JM and Riba MB, series eds). Washington, DC, American Psychiatric Press, 2000

Matchar DB, Young WB, Rosenberg JH, et al: Evidence-based guidelines for migraine headache in the primary care setting: pharmacologic management of acute attacks. 2002. Available at: http://www.aan.com/professionals/practice/pdfs/gl0087.pdf. Accessed February 26, 2007.

Mathew NT, Tietjen GE, Lucker C: Serotonin syndrome complicating migraine pharmacotherapy. Cephalalgia 16:323–327, 1996

Max MB, Lynch SA, Muir J, et al: Effects of desipramine, amitriptyline, and fluoxetine on pain in diabetic neuropathy. N Engl J Med 326:1250–1256, 1992

McEvoy G (ed): American Hospital Formulary Service (AHFS) Drug Information 2006. Bethesda, MD, American Society of Health-System Pharmacists, 2006

McLean M: Clinical pharmacokinetics of gabapentin. Neurology 44 (suppl 5):17–22, 1994

McNairy SL, Maruta T, Ivnik RJ, et al: Prescription medication dependence and neuropsychologic function. Pain 18:169–177, 1984

McQuay H, Carroll D, Jadad AR, et al: Anticonvulsant drugs for management of pain: a systematic review. BMJ 311:1047–1052, 1995

McQuay HJ, Moore RA: Methods of therapeutic trials, in Textbook of Pain, 4th Edition. Edited by Wall PD, Melzack R. Edinburgh, Churchill Livingstone, 1999, pp 1125–1138

Nemmani KVS, Mogil JS: Serotonin-GABA interactions in the modulation of mu- and kappa-opioid analgesia. Neuropharmacology 44:304–310, 2003

Novak V, Kanard R, Kissel JT, et al: Treatment of painful sensory neuropathy with tiagabine: a pilot study. Clin Auton Res 11:357–361, 2001

Pappagallo M: Newer antiepileptic drugs: possible uses in the treatment of neuropathic pain and migraine. Clin Ther 25:2506–2538, 2003

Pick CG, Paul D, Eison MS, et al: Potentiation of opioid analgesia by the antidepressant nefazodone. Eur J Pharmacol 211:375–381, 1992

Portenoy RK: Opioid therapy for chronic nonmalignant pain: a review of the critical issues. J Pain Symptom Manage 11:203–217, 1996

Portenoy RK, Hagen NA: Breakthrough pain: definition, prevalence and characteristics. Pain 41:273–281, 1990

Putnam GP, O'Quinn S, Bolden-Watson CP, et al: Migraine polypharmacy and the tolerability of sumatriptan: a large-scale, prospective study. Cephalalgia 19:668–675, 1999

Ragheb MA, Powell AL: Failure of sulindac to increase serum lithium levels. J Clin Psychiatry 47:33–34, 1986

Reissig JE, Rybarczyk AM: Pharmacologic treatment of opioid-induced sedation in chronic pain. Ann Pharmacother 39:727–731, 2005

Remillard G: Oxcarbazepine and intractable trigeminal neuralgia. Epilepsia 35:528–529, 1994

Rowbotham MC, Goli V, Kunz NR, et al: Venlafaxine extended release in the treatment of painful diabetic neuropathy: a double-blind, placebo-controlled study. Pain 110:697–706, 2004

Rumore MM, Schlichting DA: Clinical efficacy of antihistamines as analgesics. Pain 25:7–22, 1986

Samborski W, Lezanska-Szpera M, Rybakowski JK: Open trial of mirtazapine in patients with fibromyalgia. Pharmacopsychiatry 37:168–170, 2004

Sang CN, Booher S, Gilron I, et al: Dextromethorphan and memantine in painful diabetic neuropathy and postherpetic neuralgia: efficacy and dose-response trials. Anesthesiology 96:1053–1061, 2002

Saper JR, Silberstein SD, Lake AE, et al: Double-blind trial of fluoxetine: chronic daily headache and migraine. Headache 34:497–502, 1994

Saper JR, Lake AE, Tepper SJ: Nefazodone for chronic daily headache prophylaxis: an open-label study. Headache 41:465–474, 2001

Schreiber S, Backer MM, Weizman R, et al: Augmentation of opioid induced antinociception by the atypical antipsychotic drug risperidone in mice. Neurosci Lett 228:25–28, 1997

Schreiber S, Getslev V, Backer MM, et al: The atypical neuroleptics clozapine and olanzapine differ regarding their antinociceptive mechanisms and potency. Pharmacol Biochem Behav 64:75–80, 1999

Semenchuk MR, Sherman S, Davis B: Double-blind, randomized trial of bupropion SR for the treatment of neuropathic pain. Neurology 57:1583–1588, 2001

Shimoyama N, Shimoyama M, Elliott KJ, et al: D-Methadone is antinociceptive in the rat formalin test. J Pharmacol Exp Ther 283:648–652, 1997

Silberstein SD, Young WB, Hopkins MM, et al: Olanzapine in the treatment of refractory migraine and chronic daily headache. Cephalalgia 20:382–383, 2000

Sindrup SH, Jensen TS: Efficacy of pharmacological treatments of neuropathic pain: an update and effect related to mechanism of drug action. Pain 83:389–400, 1999

Sindrup SH, Gram LF, Brosen K, et al: The selective serotonin reuptake inhibitor paroxetine is effective in the treatment of diabetic neuropathy symptoms. Pain 42:135–144, 1990

Sindrup SH, Grodum E, Gram LF, et al: Concentration–response relationship in paroxetine treatment of diabetic neuropathy symptoms: a patient-blinded dose-escalation study. Ther Drug Monit 13:408–414, 1991

Sindrup SH, Bach FW, Madsen C, et al: Venlafaxine versus imipramine in painful polyneuropathy: a randomized, controlled trial. Neurology 60:1284–1289, 2003

Snow V, Weiss K, Wall EM, et al: Pharmacologic management of acute attacks of migraine and prevention of migraine headache. Ann Intern Med 137:840–849, 2002

Solaro C, Uccelli MM, Brichetto G, et al: Topiramate relieves idiopathic and symptomatic trigeminal neuralgia. J Pain Symptom Manage 21:367–368, 2001

Sommer BR, Petrides G: A case of baclofen-induced psychotic depression. J Clin Psychiatry 53:211–212, 1992

Stambaugh JE, Wainer IW: Drug interaction: meperidine and chlorpromazine, a toxic combination. J Clin Pharmacol 21:140–146, 1981

Sternbach H: The serotonin syndrome. Am J Psychiatry 148:705–713, 1991

Svendsen KB, Jensen TS, Bach FW: Does the cannabinoid dronabinol reduce central pain in multiple sclerosis? Randomised double blind placebo controlled crossover trial. BMJ 329:253–260, 2004

Swerdlow M: Anticonvulsant drugs and chronic pain. Clin Neuropharmacol 7:51–82, 1984

Taiwo YO, Fabian A, Pazoles CJ, et al: Potentiation of morphine antinociception by monoamine reuptake inhibitors in the rat spinal cord. Pain 21:329–337, 1985

Turner JA, Deyo RA, Loeser JD, et al: The importance of placebo effects in pain treatment and research. JAMA 271:1609–1614, 1994

Ventafridda V, Caraceni A, Saita L, et al: Trazodone for deafferentation pain: comparison with amitriptyline. Psychopharmacology (Berl) 95 (suppl):S44–S49, 1988

Vitton O, Gendreau M, Gendreau J, et al: A double-blind placebo-controlled trial of milnacipran in the treatment of fibromyalgia. Hum Psychopharmacol Clin Exp 19 (suppl 1):S27–S35, 2004

Weissman DE, Haddox JD: Opioid pseudoaddiction: an iatrogenic syndrome. Pain 36:363–366, 1989

Wise MG, Rundell JR: Pain and analgesics, in Clinical Manual of Psychosomatic Medicine: A Guide to Consultation-Liaison Psychiatry. Washington, DC, American Psychiatric Publishing, 2005, pp 228–229

Zakrzewska JM, Chaudhry Z, Nurmikko TJ, et al: Lamotrigine (Lamictal) in refractory trigeminal neuralgia: results from a double-blind placebo controlled crossover trial. Pain 73:223–230, 1997

Zijlstra TR, Barendregt PJ, van de Laar MAF: Venlafaxine in fibromyalgia: results of a randomized, placebo-controlled, double-blind trial (abstract). Arthritis Rheum 46 (suppl 9):S105, 2002

6

Psychotherapy

Given that pain is a multidimensional construct, a number of psychotherapeutic and adjunctive techniques may be employed to address the biological, psychological, and social features associated with and contributing to pain (Table 6–1). These interventions are not mutually exclusive but complement each other to effectively address a particular patient's needs and produce relief—that is, reducing sensory components of pain (e.g., by relaxation and hypnosis) or reducing the emotional and psychosocial distress that may accompany pain.

The psychotherapies differ with regard to their approach, perspectives, and goals. Behavior therapy is based on learning principles and holds that the patient engages in behavior(s) maintained by environmental contingencies. To modify behavior, the proactive therapist, in conjunction with others in the patient's life, modifies those contingencies to facilitate desired behaviors or extinguish problematic ones.

By contrast, psychodynamically oriented therapies are based on the perspective that the patient's behaviors are grounded in earlier developmental experiences. To understand these experiences, the therapist relies on exploration of defenses, transference, and resistance (Lakoff 1983). The patient is active, pro-

Table 6-1.   Components of pain and associated psychotherapeutic interventions

Pain component	Psychotherapeutic intervention
Biological	Relaxation training
	Biofeedback
Psychological	
Cognitive	Cognitive-behavioral therapy
	Hypnosis
Affective	Dynamically oriented therapy
	Supportive psychotherapy
Social	Behavior therapy
	Marital, couples, and family therapies
	Vocational training

ducing the material that makes up the focus of the therapeutic interventions. The therapist integrates and interprets the material brought forth in therapy, presenting it for the patient's assimilation and use. Ideally, the patient gains insight into the origins of these behaviors and then can make determinations of how to readjust current patterns of behavior to more satisfactorily meet his or her needs.

If behavior therapy and psychodynamically oriented therapies are considered to be the extreme poles of a continuum of psychotherapeutic approaches, supportive psychotherapy and cognitive-behavioral therapy (CBT) would lie somewhere along the middle. With these therapies there is no attempt to relate current behavior patterns to early developmental experiences. In supportive therapy, positive transferences are encouraged and attempts are made to bolster adaptive defenses. In contrast, CBT focuses on the patient's belief systems that are temporally related to problematic behaviors and that, when modified, bring about behavior change.

Selection of therapeutic approach depends on the patient's needs and desired goals, the resources available, and the therapist's training, skills, and preferences. Thus, if a patient presents with excessive and incapacitating use of opiate analgesics, excessive reclining, and deficiencies in self-care, the behavioral approach might be entertained. However, this approach would probably be abandoned if the therapist could not enlist the support of others with whom the patient resided to maintain the behavioral contingencies that would result in modifications of maladaptive behaviors. Dynamically oriented therapies are designed to bring about fundamental personality changes and address relationship difficulties, but these therapies might well be abandoned if the patient is not psychologically minded or is in a terminal condition in which life expectancy could prove to be prohibitive. CBT could be more desirable in such situations, but it would be abandoned if the patient could not modify cognitive strategies encompassing his or her worldview and, similarly, coping strategies because of intervening cognitive disorders.

Resistance to Psychotherapy

Among patients with complex pain, there can be several challenges to the prospect of psychotherapy. Such patients have a history of medical disappointments and could well be frustrated with health care providers. As a consequence, these patients might believe there is no relief on the horizon. They could be angry, suspicious, and defensive, and they may possibly reject psychological interventions (Stieg et al. 1999).

To have the patient align with the therapist and learn the work of psychotherapy, the therapist needs to establish an atmosphere of safety. The therapist needs to facilitate an understanding of the processes involved in the therapy by educating the patient about the role of therapy and what the patient can come to expect from the work of therapy in addressing pain-related issues. A particular mechanism might involve emphasizing the empowerment that may be derived from therapy. Although the variables in an individual's life—and in particular, pain—are not all entirely under his or her direct control, patients may be able to effect changes—within the range of their abilities—and take control of their lives. The therapist is instrumental in forging the therapeutic alliance and a working relationship.

For some patients, being proactive in effecting life changes can be a stirring and stimulating prospect, empowering them to take charge of their lives, pain, quality of life, and destinies. For others, this prospect can be frightening and one to be avoided at all cost. The therapist needs to address such ambivalences in the context of the early work in therapy.

Some patients are more amenable to effecting life changes than others. Such changes may include making efforts to reduce medication use or misuse, increasing physical activity, increasing social participation, returning to productive activity, undertaking weight loss, or addressing nicotine, alcohol, or substance abuse cessation. Patient readiness for the rehabilitation changes required in chronic pain can be conceived of in several stages (Prochaska and DiClemente 1983). Some persons are not at all ready to effect life changes or see no need for lifestyle modifications (i.e., are in the precontemplation stage). Others might be ambivalent about making such changes but feel that they lack insight into how to go about making them (the contemplation stage). Patients in the contemplation stage may benefit from education about and exploration of the impact of pain on current life patterns. Following the contemplation stage is the preparation stage, in which a patient begins to make efforts to effect change; then come the action and maintenance stages, in which the patient, with the assistance of the therapist and others in his or her life, employs strategies to effect changes and maintains the modifications in behavior while avoiding lapses to less effective coping and behavioral strategies.

Resistance to therapy may be overcome by engaging the patient with chronic pain. First, the therapist must accept the pain at face value rather than try to ascertain its validity or establish its somatic origins. The therapist's focus should be on the patient's subjective experience of pain and the impact of that pain on the patient's life. Second, education of the patient about the bridge between psychological factors and pain might be required. Finally, the therapist may enlist the patient by emphasizing that the goals of therapy can empower the patient by facilitating growth, coping, adaptation, and so forth.

Factors to Be Addressed in Psychotherapy

Regardless of the psychotherapeutic approach undertaken, there are certain essential psychological components of the pain experience that are likely to be the focus of therapy. Some of these might be more central to a particular psychotherapeutic approach than others.

Affect

Chronic pain is associated with a wide range of psychosocial problems, including strained relationships, alienation from others, problems with depression and anger, and loss experiences (e.g., bodily integrity, self-efficacy). The psychological experiences of patients with chronic pain may include significant mood disturbances. These in turn may have an impact on thought patterns and belief systems, all of which may profoundly influence the pain experience and the extent to which patients adapt to their condition, adhere to treatment, and participate in the work of rehabilitation.

Little can be done to facilitate rehabilitation and restoration of functioning unless comorbid mood disorders are addressed and treated. Given that the neurophysiology and neuroanatomy of pain processing pathways overlap with those of affective processing and experience, pain perception and mood states (e.g., depression and anxiety) have mutually reciprocal relationships. Thus, affective states may influence pain perception, pain reporting, and pain-related behaviors. For example, the severity of a patient's depressive symptoms has been shown to predict the number and severity of pain complaints (Hawley and Wolfe 1988). Depression is a significant predictor of average daily pain (Affleck et al. 1991).

The experience and expression of anger may have an impact on chronic pain. Higher levels of anger (as well as depression and anxiety) are found among patients with chronic low back pain than are found among asymptomatic control subjects (Feuerstein 1986). Poorly managed anger adversely affects pain levels. In one study, patients with chronic tension headache differed from control subjects in their experience and expression of anger (Hatch et al. 1991). Headache patients were prone to hostility (i.e., feelings of resentment, suspicion, and mistrust), anger arousal (i.e., perceiving situations as annoying or frustrating and aroused to anger frequently), and anger suppression (i.e., being more likely to suppress angry feelings once aroused). However, once overtly angry, headache patients tended to expend less control over the expression of anger than control subjects. Taken together, these studies suggest that modulation of anger and hostility might be a major determinant of the experience of certain chronic pain conditions (Burns 1997).

In the context of psychotherapy, a patient's unpleasant emotions may be focused on to reduce distress. Emotions—including anger—contain information value. The patient can become empowered by using the information gleaned from these emotions. So, for anger, the emotion might serve as a signal that one's rights have been violated, one's needs are not being met, an injustice has been done, or one is compromising oneself. Recognizing this, patients may possibly expend less energy suppressing anger and instead engage in measures such as determining how their needs are not being met and what action to take. The experience of anger is likely to contribute to physical discomfort when there is a conflict around the expression of anger and there are high levels of hostility.

Table 6–2. Psychotherapy interventions employed to facilitate access of emotions

Help patients to

    Identify and label feelings.

    Recognize affect as a signal.

    Identify the precipitant for the feelings.

    Express feelings with words instead of actions (e.g., substance abuse, excessive narcotic use, suicide gestures).

    Reduce anhedonia.

    Take better care of themselves.

Determine what can be done with unpleasant feelings (e.g., use judicious expression of emotions, take constructive action).

Psychotherapy may be particularly useful in assisting patients with pain to manage unpleasant emotional states. The basic approach is outlined in Table 6–2. However, the approaches differ. Psychodynamically oriented approaches might consider how emotions were dealt with and managed earlier in development. The strategy invoked is to demonstrate how such approaches, when employed in adulthood, are ineffective in producing growth. CBT, on the other hand, is more focused on here-and-now experiences, problem solving, and development of effective coping strategies.

Factors that contribute to impairments in regulating emotions are outlined in Table 6–3. Certain disorders—for example, posttraumatic stress disorder and dissociative and somatoform disorders—are characterized by an inability to access emotions, leading to affective blunting, somatic amplification, or both. Even among pain patients without comorbid Axis I disorders, there may be a propensity to employ defenses (e.g., isolation of affect and alexithymia) that shield them from intolerable emotions (Beutler et al. 1986).

Defenses

Early psychodynamic conceptualizations of pain emphasized that the symptoms of pain serve a function (see Table 6–4), such as allowing one to cope with unpleasant emotions, allowing one to enlist the support of others, or serving as a way to expiate guilt. Such conceptualizations have been difficult to corroborate empirically (Weisberg and Keefe 1999) but nonetheless illustrate that conflicts and defenses against those conflicts may have an impact on the experience of pain.

Table 6–3. Reasons why emotions are poorly identified and regulated

Patient fears that if emotions are expressed
  He or she will be abandoned.
  The emotions (experienced as intense states) might lead to some catastrophic result (e.g., rage-filled reaction).
Patient has not learned that emotions can be expressed appropriately.
Patient has not had good role models for the effective expression of emotion (e.g., had parent who had tantrums).
Patient is unable to access emotions because of posttraumatic stress disorder, dissociative disorders, personality disorders, or substance abuse disorders.
Patient is using emotional defenses (e.g., isolation of affect, alexithymia).

Defenses serve to reduce the access of intolerable affective states or impulses from awareness. For example, if a person cannot tolerate an unpleasant emotion (e.g., anger), he or she might project that emotion onto others (e.g., the therapist), leading to potential disruptions in relationships (e.g., the doctor–patient relationship). Primitive defenses might also include projective identification, whereby the patient enlists the object onto whom he or she has projected to act out the patient's aggressive impulses. Such strategies may potentially undermine relationships and exasperate available support systems. Additional defenses accompanying chronic pain include denial, reaction formation, and repression (Tauschke et al. 1990).

Table 6–4. Early psychodynamic conceptualizations of pain

Proponent	Concept
Freud (1893)	Psychological distress is expressed through somatic complaints. Chronic pain is similar to mourning.
Szasz (1957)	Pain serves a symbolic function for emotions that are difficult to tolerate and therefore remain unexpressed.
	Pain diverts attention away from the emotion and underlying conflict.
	Pain provides one with a basis for seeking assistance from others.
Engel (1959)	Pain serves to
	Absolve one from guilt.
	Distract one from aggressive impulses.
	Rationalize failure and justify one's persistent perception of being defeated.

Patients with chronic pain may have deficits in self-regulation brought on by difficulties in managing affect and behavior. For example, alexithymia, present among those who demonstrate asymbolic and concrete thinking, is characterized by the patient's inability to identify and communicate feeling states (Krystal 1982). Just as often, the person's feelings are vague, ill defined, and confusing. These factors may lead to impairments in self-regulation that could bring about generalized states of distress and acting out in ways that undermine treatment, disturb relationships, and exacerbate life problems. For example, intense feelings may be temporarily dissipated in several ways: by focusing on pain (instead of the unpleasant emotion), through use of analgesics that can produce changes in one's emotional states (e.g., opiates), and through abuse of substances.

In examining the therapist–patient relationship, the therapist can be aware of the defenses employed and can redirect the patient's attention to the problematic emotions that may be underlying the defense. As with addressing unpleasant emotional states, the goals of therapy may be to assist the patient with identifying the utility of his or her defenses, replacing destructive or primitive defenses, and substituting healthier defenses (e.g., humor, sublimation).

A number of higher-level defenses may be employed in the management of unpleasant emotional states. Of these, humor can be quite effective. Patients who are humorless are prone to being overwhelmed by the ordinary vicissitudes of life. Similarly, loss of humor among those enlisted to assist in the care of the patient might signal impending burnout. In experimental paradigms, individuals exposed to painful stimuli had greater pain tolerability when exposed to laughter-inducing tapes than persons who used distracting mental tasks (e.g., calculating mental arithmetic) or those who were not given any instruction about strategies to use with regard to tolerating pain (Cogan et al. 1987).

A question arises as to whether laughter is the same as humor. Laughter is really a reaction to a laughter-provoking event, whereas humor is a defense employed to diffuse the emotional valence of one's actions. Humor is a mechanism of distancing oneself from life stressors, examining one's own actions, and so forth. Nonetheless, the utility of humor with regard to pain has been long advocated.

Belief Systems and Cognitive Distortions

One's beliefs can have an impact on pain, treatment, and response to treatment. Belief systems (or schemata) are of three major types. One type includes belief systems that are broad and encompass aspects and beliefs about one's life, world, relationships, and so forth. The second type comprises those belief systems that are considered to be more stable, influencing one's relationships, work ethic, and manner of relating to others—these would be commensurate with personality characteristics. The third type includes belief systems that are more or less specific to the pain experience. The stable beliefs affecting personality style as well as those pertaining specifically to pain are likely to influence coping and adaptation to the entire pain experience. They can be evaluated by various assessment techniques (DeGood and Tait 2001) and might become some of the grist for the mill in psychotherapeutic interventions. These beliefs can affect coping strategies and are likely to be of relevance in interventions such as cognitive-behavioral, dynamic, and supportive therapies. A person with a grin-and-bear-it schema would approach pain brought on by physical therapy differently from the person who views pain as reflecting a serious pathologic state. For the latter patient, activity might be construed as dangerous. A person who believes that pain is equivalent to disability may be more inclined to neglect usual responsibilities than one who does not.

Expectations and beliefs about treatment are likewise likely to have an impact on a person's response to pain and on a patient's treatment adherence. Thus, the patient's perception of his or her role (e.g., proactive, informed, and instrumental versus passive, uninformed, and dependent on the physician's interventions) will likely affect treatment adherence and willingness to explore possible treatment interventions. Similarly, the patient might have expectations about the role of the physician and others involved in the multidisciplinary treatment of pain. A patient's expectation might be that to be effective, a treatment must entirely alleviate pain and discomfort. In reality, however, a more plausible approach might be to expect some relief along with improved adaptation and quality of life. For some patients, such improvements can fall short of expectations. Some patients see the role of treatment to be exclusively medically based, whereas others might be amenable to recognizing that psychological variables can, and often do, reduce pain and improve life quality. Similarly, expectations of treatment outcome are likely to have an impact on one's expectations of recovery, rehabilitation, and restoration of function.

Belief systems can arise from one's early developmental experiences, earlier life experiences, earlier experiences with the medical community (either direct or indirect through the medical encounters shared with others who were ill), and relationships with others. Beliefs shape expectations, not only about recovery and rehabilitation but also about what one can expect out of life in general (e.g., shaping one's sense of future hope versus helplessness). Such belief systems influence how one views oneself, shaping one's sense of self-efficacy, autonomy, and self-esteem (Seligman 1990).

In addition to belief systems, the patient's cognitive styles and propensity toward cognitive distortions (see also Chapter 3, "Evaluation of the Pain Patient," of this book) are likely to reduce self-efficacy, hamper development of effective coping, drain the patient's support systems, accentuate unpleasant emotional states (e.g., anger, anxiety, depression), and exacerbate pain. For example, catastrophizing (i.e., the tendency to view and expect the worst in response to pain) has been seen as a cognitive approach that may predispose one to heightened pain (Sullivan et al. 1998). Cognitive distortions such as this can be determined, or at least influenced, by mood states (e.g., depression, anxiety). Because depression often coexists with unremitting pain, it becomes difficult to determine whether catastrophizing is a result of pain and predisposes one to depression, or whether pain and comorbid depression result in a tendency to catastrophize.

Catastrophizing may consist of three distinct cognitive distortions: rumination, magnification, and helplessness (Sullivan et al. 1995). The clinician's identification of these distortions, ascertained by careful clinical inquiry (see also Chapter 3 of this book) and perhaps by use of assessment scales, could be pivotal to understanding the psychological, emotional, and other disabling aspects of pain. The goal of cognitive-behavioral strategies is to address these distortions. When these distortions are altered, the patient may more effectively cope, may experience less emotional distress, and may overcome some of the disabling aspects of the pain.

Behavior Therapy

The goal of behavior therapy is to mitigate excessive problematic pain-associated behaviors (e.g., excessive medication usage, limping) and increase those adaptive behaviors occurring infrequently or not at all (e.g., walking, exercise, self-care, work) (Sanders 2003). The steps involved in behavior therapy are outlined in Table 6–5. As originally described, behavior therapy was conducted with patients with chronic pain on an inpatient basis (Fordyce et al. 1982).

Table 6–5. Steps of behavior therapy

Step 1: Define problem behaviors (operants) that warrant attention (e.g., medication use, excessive reclining, avoidance of activities).

Step 2: Determine the relationship between operants and environmental consequences (i.e., identify reinforcers and the temporal contingencies that exist to maintain these).

Step 3: Assess whether the link between operants and reinforcers is modifiable (i.e., identify whether reinforcers can be modified so that they become contingent on desired [adaptive] behaviors, identify how frequently reinforcers should be applied after desired behaviors occur, identify what quotas might need to be established, identify those persons who should be involved in the contingency management process [e.g., spouse, significant other]).

Step 4: Establish how the systematic disruption of problem behaviors and consequences can be conducted (i.e., how to extinguish undesired behaviors [which reinforcers should be withheld and when]).

Step 5: Establish transferability to home and work (i.e., consider to what extent the contingencies can be translated into the home, work, or any setting in which it becomes necessary to maintain these desired behaviors; perform follow-up assessments; determine if contingencies need to be modified in other settings; determine if the newly learned behaviors have been extinguished and whether these can be reinstated).

Source. Adapted from Fordyce WE, Roberts AH, Sternbach RA: "The Behavioral Management of Chronic Pain: A Response to Critics." *Pain* 22:113–125, 1985. Copyright 1985, International Association for the Study of Pain. Used with permission.

The therapy was highly structured by the therapist and treating staff. In outpatient settings, however, behavior therapy is obviously less well controlled. The assistance of others is needed to ensure that environmental contingencies are systematically applied at home or in other relevant settings.

Behavior therapy is predicated on the recognition that the events (consequences) following a behavior will influence the extent to which that behavior is likely to recur. Simply put, behaviors that are followed by pleasant or desirable consequences (reinforcements) are likely to be repeated in the future, whereas those followed by negative consequences are not likely to recur. There are two types of reinforcement: positive and negative. Positive reinforcement increases the likelihood of a target (i.e., desired) behavior by providing a positive, pleasant, or desired consequence. On the other hand, negative reinforcement increases the likelihood of a target (desired) behavior by removing an unpleasant consequence. Behavior change is brought about by active modification of the consequences that follow the patient's behavior. Reinforcement can include something given to the person—for example, attention, praise, or the chance to do something the patient finds rewarding (e.g., rest, reading, watching a favorite television program). A contingency might be established that if the patient walks 200 feet, the patient is rewarded with the opportunity to watch a favored 30-minute television program. Quotas might be set for greater distances over time, upon which reinforcement would be contingent (Fordyce et al. 1985).

Undesirable behaviors are those that interfere with adaptive functioning (e.g., excessive medication use; avoidance of rehabilitative measures, leading to generalized deconditioning). Undesirable behaviors can be extinguished by modifying the consequences. When the reinforcers that normally follow these behaviors are withheld, the behavior is less likely to recur. Alternatively, aversive consequences (e.g., punishment) can be applied following the behavior and are likely to reduce the likelihood of recurrence. In behavior therapy, punishments are not employed to modify problematic pain-related behaviors. There are several drawbacks to the use of punishment (e.g., the patient engages in these behaviors when the "punisher" is not around to notice). Consequently, withholding of consequences that would customarily reinforce undesirable behaviors is the preferred approach.

Critics of behavior therapy argue that the behavioral modifications might not be sustained. Setbacks may occur once the desired outcome is achieved or the incentive is gone. Alternative reinforcers (e.g., praise, attention) may need to be set in place to maintain the behaviors. The behavioral changes can dissipate in settings (e.g., home, work) in which reinforcement patterns are less systematic or consistent. In addition, despite the changes acquired in behavior therapy, the patient may nonetheless experience pain—what is modified is the overt behavior, not the perception of pain.

Critics also argue that the behavioral approach is simplistic—specifically, the idea that the person engages in behavior because he or she comes to expect a particular outcome. Thus, behavior therapy fails to factor in those qualities of being human that influence and dictate behavior. For example, expectation, anticipation, thinking, planning, and remembering can also influence behavior and mediate pain-related behavior and perception (Seligman 1990).

As an illustration, passivity and inactivity can be particularly problematic in a variety of pain states (e.g., low back pain, arthritis). This lack of activity can result in generalized deconditioning, muscle weakness, and reduced endurance—all of which can exacerbate pain once an effort is undertaken. From a behavioral perspective, such passivity might be reinforced by others (e.g., a spouse who engages in solicitous behaviors and tends to the patient's needs once the inactivity is noticed). An alternative explanation might attribute the inactivity or restricted activity to expectations the patient has that activity will exacerbate pain. Thus, the patient is avoiding the prospect of pain, a factor that may be more pivotal in determining the inactivity. Yet another explanation suggests that passivity arises from the patient's belief that what he or she does is pointless (i.e., learned helplessness), so why bother to walk, exercise, and so forth. Thus, the cognitive-behavioral approach has been invoked to address problematic behaviors by taking into account the cognitive aspects of the patient that might dictate such behaviors.

Cognitive-Behavioral Therapy

CBT addresses the correction of distorted thinking processes and the development of strategies (coping) with which to deal effectively with pain, its effects, and psychosocial stressors. CBT has been applied to a number of different chronic pain problems, including low back pain, headache, fibromyalgia, osteoarthritis, rheumatoid arthritis, and temporomandibular joint disorders (Turner and Chapman 1982a). Empirical evidence suggests that CBT is as effective in facilitating psychological adjustment and reducing reported pain levels as standard medical treatment conditions (Compas et al. 1998; Keefe et al. 1992; Morley et al. 1999). However, when return to work was assessed among patients with low back pain specifically, CBT was found to be no more effective than control situations (Scheer et al. 1997).

CBT focuses on internal appraisals of pain and disability by examining and addressing the cognitions, emotions, and behaviors associated with pain and pain-related activities. Conducted in about 8–12 fifty-minute sessions, the therapy is structured, with clear agendas set by the patient and therapist focusing on prominent areas of concern for the patient. The therapist is directive, guiding the use of homework treatments, outlining exercises, and assessing the efficacy of the modalities employed, yet this role remains flexible, with the patient's input guiding any shifts undertaken in the therapy. CBT assumes a collaborative effort between the patient and therapist (Fishman and Loscalzo 1987).

The model for understanding the approach of CBT is illustrated in Figure 6–1. In this model, disturbed emotional and behavioral responses are a direct function of specific maladaptive cognitions (i.e., one's beliefs, expectations, and thought processes). These in turn lead to an array of physiologic changes that can precipitate or exacerbate pain. CBT emphasizes modification of maladaptive cognitions and beliefs (schemata) and the development of effective coping strategies. CBT provides patients with direction and instruction to reappraise thoughts and events occurring in their life experiences. Faulty appraisals and misattributions are reframed and replaced with those that are reality-based (i.e., less irrational). The presumption, then, is that there will be less physiologic arousal occurring within the patient. This diminished arousal in turn would be less apt to accentuate the individual's pain experiences.

In CBT, it is recognized that the patient often cannot control or avoid distressing life events. However, the patient can almost always exert some control over how much distress, suffering, and life disruption those events produce. This control can be achieved by altering one's perceptions of these events, their significance, and their meaning, and by altering one's coping. Unlike in other psychotherapeutic approaches, external contingencies of reward, internal dispositions, and acquired developmental processes are de-emphasized.

The patients with the best long-term results are those who apply CBT skills learned in session to real-life situations. In these sessions, homework is required. This homework entails keeping a diary (much like the pain diary described in Chapter 3 of this book), in which the patient records his or her levels of pain in different situations, along with feelings and thoughts occurring at the time. Homework assignments, if completed properly, help the patient and therapist identify those situations, moods, feelings, and thought processes associated with pain. This process then highlights the points of interventions to work on in therapy (i.e., which cognitions require restructuring and when to employ coping strategies).

Cognitive restructuring, an interactive process involving the Socratic method, is used to teach patients to identify and modify maladaptive, negatively distorted thoughts that may lead to negative feelings, such as depression, anxiety, and anger. The patient is encouraged to examine irrational, self-defeating thoughts and discriminate between these and more rational alternatives. For patients with pain, emotional reactions to pain can be greatly influenced by thoughts. Coping skills training is aimed at helping patients develop a reper-

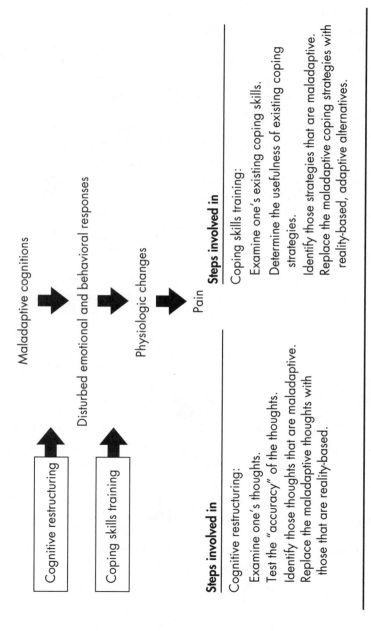

Figure 6–1. Modalities involved in cognitive-behavioral therapy.

toire of skills for managing pain and stress and providing patients with a general set of problem-solving or coping skills that can be used in a wide range of situations that induce pain.

Coping refers to the strategies used by the person to deal with the pain and life stressors (Weickgenant et al. 1993). The strategies employed are based on how the person appraises a given situation or life event. Components of appraisal include the value or significance the person assigns to the event, the perception of the impact of the event, and the assessment of the resources the person believes himself or herself to have with which to deal with the event.

The diversity and range of coping strategies employed might signal that the patient's repertoire of dealing with pain and its effects on his or her life requires modification. Ineffective coping may possibly be associated with psychiatric disturbances such as depression. For example, depressed patients with low back pain were found to be restricted in the range and types of coping strategies they used when compared with nondepressed patients with low back pain (Weickgenant et al. 1993). The therapist helps the patient develop a broader range of effective coping strategies by examining existing coping strategies, determining their effectiveness, and facilitating the development of a broader range of strategies. Different strategies may need to be employed in different settings, and patients may need assistance in deciphering which strategies would be most effective.

Active coping can involve developing problem-solving strategies (e.g., problem-focused coping, social support seeking). By contrast, passive coping involves internal self-statements that the patient learns to say to him- or herself to facilitate coping and might include wishful thinking, self-blame, and avoidance. For example, depressed patients with low back pain were inclined to be less productive and to employ passive coping strategies when dealing with life stressors, whereas nondepressed patients with low back pain employed active coping strategies. However, the latter group did employ passive coping strategies when attempting to deal with the pain experience (Weickgenant et al. 1993). Coping then may be either problem focused or emotion focused.

To help patients modify coping strategies, the therapist should identify currently employed strategies, assess the utility of these strategies (whether they facilitate the patient's relief), and point out, develop, and refine alternatives. Thus, the patient who tends to employ passive strategies, such as self-blame and avoidance, might be encouraged to develop strategies that are more active and self-soothing.

CBT has the advantage of broad applicability in a number of situations. It is a relatively low-cost intervention and appears to be cost-effective. On the other hand, CBT has the disadvantage of requiring sustained active patient participation. Also, therapists need to have specialized training in CBT in order to use it effectively.

Supportive Therapy

Much of what clinicians do can be considered under the auspices of supportive psychotherapy. For the patient with chronic or complex pain, complete pain relief might not be possible; supportive therapy might then be a viable approach. The therapist should undertake a warm, reflective, and empathic approach to reduce patient distress and reassure the patient that he or she is understood and that the magnitude of his or her plight is appreciated. Feedback should be given, providing patients with the outcome and findings of physical and laboratory assessments, pain assessments, and psychometric testing. Rather than telling the patient that "nothing can be done," the therapist should emphasize that modification and improvement in functioning are essentially the patient's responsibility. This emphasis can enhance the patient's sense of personal control and self-efficacy, which is critical for overcoming the tendency of the patient to succumb to powerlessness and helplessness. Therapists may offer a menu of concrete advice for strategies to reduce discomfort, improve sleep, address medication use, and develop pain-modulating interventions (e.g., relaxation training). Such a menu fosters the notion of the patient's responsibility and autonomy by allowing the patient to select those aspects of treatment that are most appealing, thus possibly facilitating patient compliance (Miller and Sanchez 1994).

Ongoing follow-up with supportive therapy is required. The interventions described above will be most successful when subsequent meetings with the patient allow for repeated interventions. In addition, setbacks may be the basis for determining what modifications in medications and other treatment interventions might be required. Follow-up reinforces the notion that the patient and physician or clinician are working in concert to effectively mitigate pain and optimize adaptive functioning while restoring pleasure and balance and bolstering relationships in the patient's life. With this reinforcement, the patient can avoid the potential pitfall of viewing himself or herself as passive and helpless in the treatment process.

Marital, Couples, and Family Therapy

Pain is often myopically viewed as an individual patient's problem. Painful disorders have an impact on a broader spectrum of persons, including the patient's partner and family, along with friendships and work relationships. Conversely, social factors may contribute to the onset, exacerbation, maintenance, and course of the pain disorder.

Significant changes in the functioning and activity of the family unit can arise as a result of having a member with pain. These changes can include alterations in the role responsibilities within the home in order to assume those that the pain patient is no longer able to perform. Such role modifications may be emotionally laden, with some members feeling burdened and the patient experiencing loss of self-efficacy or feeling as though he or she is viewed as incapable. There also may be resulting shifts of influence and decision making within the home.

Several stressors may affect the patient's relationships. One such stressor may be related to financial issues, such as lost employment, treatment costs, and inadequate medical coverage. The patient and partner (along with other family members) may disagree about the feasibility of return to work or exploration of other vocational pursuits.

Another stressor may involve the reactions of others to the patient's pain. The reactions of persons within the home can be quite varied, including solicitous responses, withdrawal, and indifference. The solicitous spouse or significant other of the patient might inadvertently reinforce pain complaints and related pain behaviors (e.g., grimacing, limping, sighing) by eagerly accommodating the patient when such behaviors are expressed. Some studies have demonstrated that the degree of solicitous behavior on the part of one's partner is an important factor in determining or predicting pain reports (Block et al. 1980).

Patients also vary in their response to others' reactions. They may harbor expectations of how the partner (or others within the family) should respond to their pain complaints and pain-related behaviors. They may view such responses negatively (e.g., as demeaning or indicative of the patient's "invalid" status), or they may view them as supportive and helpful.

Strained communication patterns within the couple or family may be another stressor. Direct discussion of the patient's behavior may be difficult. The pain may serve as a means of avoiding discussion about particular topics, which leads to unresolved conflicts and emotional difficulties. Sexual dysfunction and a decline in intimacy from prepain periods may add to the burden of the patient and his or her partner as well. Formal sex therapy may be needed, especially when such difficulties foreshadow more deleterious effects on the relationship.

Another potential stressor is that normal interests (e.g., in outside hobbies and activities) may no longer be available to the patient, partner, or other family members. Social support networks that would normally be relied on might be less accessible. The patient and his or her primary caregivers may have little emotional reserve remaining to support and care for others within the family.

As a result of any or all of these factors, the partner–patient dyad and family relationships as a whole can experience marked strain as a result of the pain disorder. Thus, marital and family therapy can be useful to address these issues, mitigating the strain experienced by the patient and others in the patient's life (Romano and Schmaling 2001). Cohesive family relationships and a supportive, mutual, and intimate relationship with a partner can be a buffer against depression for the pain patient. In addition, pain patients in such relationships tend to respond best to treatment and have lower levels of disability (Kerns and Haythornthwaite 1988; Kerns and Turk 1984).

Despite the difficulties that can afflict couples in which pain is prominent, such couples typically remain together for long periods of time. One possible explanation is that the pain serves the role of preserving homeostasis within a troubled relationship. External pressures (e.g., how others would interpret divorce or separation when one partner is so ill) may also influence why some couples remain together. Financial factors can prove to be prohibitive for one or both parties, especially when disability interferes with work functioning and financial support. Substantial financial gains could be hoped for through pending litigation, which might mean that the well partner would want to hold out for a piece of the expected financial gain. Interestingly, partners may also come to endorse significant pain problems of their own as well. Often, there is overlap of this pain in location and quality with the pain reported by the patient (Sholevar and Perkel 1990).

Assessment scales and questionnaires can augment the information gleaned from clinical interview. For example, the Multidimensional Pain Inventory, mentioned in Chapter 3 ("Evaluation of the Pain Patient") of this book, has a portion devoted to analyzing the partner's responses to pain. Other assessment instruments that assess relationship satisfaction and the family environment are available as well. Such instruments can be quite helpful when attempting to address issues arising in the social milieu of the pain patient (Romano and Schmaling 2001).

Group Therapy

One of the most devastating effects of chronic pain can be the isolation it produces for the patient. Group therapy, including self-help groups, can serve to diffuse the sense of isolation experienced by the pain patient. These groups allow for the mutual sharing of experiences, provide an opportunity to learn from the experiences of others, foster education about treatment strategies, and foster coping strategies. The shared experiences of persons in the group can offer the patient a sense of being fully understood, often without the requirement of having to explain his or her experiences or emotions to others who do not share the same level of physical pain.

Some groups are exclusive—that is, organized around particular disorders (e.g., groups for persons with fibromyalgia, arthritis, or cancer pain). Others can be inclusive—broader and open to persons with recurrent or chronic pain of various sorts. Some groups are open to family members and significant others as well.

The purposes of group therapy include reducing feelings of isolation (i.e., universalization) and providing a forum in which mutual support, information exchange, advice, modeling of effective coping, and abreaction of emotional experiences are possible. The structure of the group sets the stage for and dictates the focus and perspective of the participants. For the group to be effective, the rules of the group process need to be delineated early. If patients are allowed to ventilate distress and can respond to the support and advice offered by peers, attendance in therapy sessions can be a source of inspiration and empowerment. A special benefit arising from group process is *abreaction,* whereby repressed, emotionally laden experiences are brought to conscious awareness (i.e., reexperienced) and in the process, insight is gained. Some members of the group can inspire others with hope or the means to effectively address emotional-psychological consequences associated with the pain experience (Keefe et al. 1996).

Psychotherapeutic goals can be organized around exploring individual psychodynamics and bringing about personality change. Self-help groups, on the other hand, have vastly different goals—for example, fostering emotional well-being—and focus on coping with specific life problems. Groups vary as to whether they are organized around a particular philosophy or approach. For example, some groups have actually adapted the 12-step program originated within Alcoholics Anonymous, substituting pain for alcohol (Back and Neck Injury 2002). The goals of such programs are to view pain as something one might not be able to fully control or remove. Thus, adaptations in a person's life might be required to overcome the many obstacles in life, relationships, and spiritual life.

Adjunctive Interventions

Adjunctive interventions are not forms of therapy but are nonetheless helpful techniques that can be undertaken with the pain patient. These techniques can complement other medical treatments and psychotherapies.

Biofeedback

Biofeedback refers to a procedure in which physical parameters (e.g., muscle tension) are continuously monitored and fed back to the patient, who then attempts to alter the physical parameter. For example, an individual attempting to regulate and modify the degree of muscle tension in forehead muscles would have electromyographic electrodes placed on the forehead. The electrical signals from these electrodes would be relayed to a monitor and presented in any of a number of formats (e.g., visual, auditory). The patient, attending to the signal, would then use the information presented to develop strategies to reduce muscle tension. The principle relies on the idea that the patient uses the feedback signal as an indicator of the degree of physical activity that can be modified. In pain management, the idea is that the physical parameter measured and ideally altered is somehow linked to the genesis of pain (Turk et al. 1979; Turner and Chapman 1982b).

Various biofeedback procedures, focusing on selected physiologic parameters for selected pain states, may be employed. Thus, biofeedback from electromyography assists the patient in learning to reduce muscle tension; the levels of measured muscle tension are signaled back to the patient for modification.

This technique is useful in tension headache, temporomandibular joint disorders, fibromyalgia, and other myofascial pain disorders. Thermal biofeedback monitors skin temperature to give the patient an indicator of the degree of peripheral vasodilation. The cooler the skin, the greater the vascular constriction; this reflects the amount of prevailing sympathetic activity. By increasing the skin temperature, one is able to suppress the extent of sympathetic activity. This approach has been used in the treatment of migraine and sympathetically maintained pain. Electroencephalography has also been linked with biofeedback. Brain electrical activity is fed back to the patient and is subject to modification by the patient. The goal is to achieve states of alpha rhythm brain activity that reflect a state of relaxation. Customarily, electroencephalographic biofeedback is quite cumbersome and is not regularly used in pain treatment settings.

The technology involved in biofeedback has enhanced the opportunities and approaches available in pain management. Eventually, with practice, the patient learns to attend to physical cues that signal that relaxation, deep breathing, and changes in cognitive strategies are required (e.g., sensing one's own heightened muscle tension). The patient is then able to invoke those strategies to reduce the tension without requiring the use of the biofeedback equipment. However, some practitioners question the utility of biofeedback and the necessity of all the cumbersome technology, arguing that other strategies (e.g., relaxation training) are equally efficacious (Silver and Blanchard 1978).

Relaxation and Imagery Training

Relaxation and imagery (R&I) has been employed in both acute and chronic pain and has been successfully implemented in the treatment of tension headache, migraine headache, temporomandibular joint pain, chronic back pain, and myofascial pain syndrome (Turner and Chapman 1982a). Progressive muscle relaxation (PMR) is the most common approach used. In PMR, the patient is instructed to tense muscles in a region of the body or a limb and then subsequently relax those muscles. The tension and subsequent relaxation of muscle groups is conducted in a logical and sequential manner, generally from head to foot or the reverse. For some patients (e.g., those with myofascial pain and fibromyalgia), the process of tensing sequential muscle groups could prove to be too difficult or fatiguing. Consequently, alternative measures can be employed (e.g., guided imagery or deep breathing exercises).

Autogenic training is similar to PMR in that the patient focuses on sequential and progressive relaxation of parts of the body, but the step of tensing muscles in those regions is not required. Instead, the patient is asked to focus on sensations of heaviness and warmth extending throughout the body.

Guided imagery involves talking the patient through vivid images that are particularly comforting and relaxing. Just as imagining the taste and aroma of a craved meal or an erotic thought can induce a dramatic constellation of physiologic responses, so too, it is thought, can guided imagery modify physiologic reactions to pain. The patient is asked to imagine a place that he or she finds most relaxing in order to set the stage for being in an emotional state that would be inconsistent with anxiety or tension. The patient is then guided to vividly recapture as much of the imagined place as possible—the sights, the sounds, smells, tastes, and physical sensations and feelings. Guided imagery has been employed successfully in postsurgical and chronic pain conditions (Daake and Gueldner 1989; Mannix et al. 1999).

Deep breathing exercises involve the direction of deep breathing in a manner that potentiates a deepened relaxation. A script for deep breathing exercises is provided in Table 6–6. The patient is instructed in deep breathing so that the technique can be used at home. The technique can be used in a matter of few seconds or over a span of several minutes (McCaffery and Beebe 1999).

R&I offers several clinical advantages. It is easy for clinicians to learn how to implement R&I, and it is easily learned by patients as well. Unlike biofeedback, R&I requires no specialized equipment. At most, patients might require a tape or compact disc player to practice R&I; thus it is a low-cost intervention. Patients may be more receptive to R&I compared with other interventions, such as hypnosis, about which there may be misconceptions.

R&I has several disadvantages. It is not a sufficient treatment for pain states. Adverse effects may arise, including muscle cramping and fatigue, particularly with the use of PMR. Lack of patient practice at home limits its usefulness. In addition, certain patients might find it difficult to gain any benefit from R&I. Highly distressed or distractible patients might have marked difficulty concentrating on the techniques required. In addition, patients distracted by intense, severe pain might find that they are unable to benefit from R&I. Some religious patients and those who are rigid or concrete in their thinking might be resistant to R&I, fearing that it invokes practices contrary to their spiritual experiences or cognitive styles. (This resistance can generally

Table 6–6.   Script for deep breathing exercises

Have the patient assume a comfortable position in a quiet place where there will be no interruptions. Ask the patient to imagine that he or she is doing this exercise in a place that is calming and relaxing. Then, instruct the patient as follows:

1.   Breathe in slowly and deeply.
2.   As you breathe out slowly, feel yourself beginning to relax as tension begins to leave your body.
3.   Now, breathe in and out regularly and slowly. Constrict your abdominal muscles, and feel your chest wall expand as your abdomen compresses inward. Feel your ribs expand, hold this, then slowly release. As you release the air, feel your body relax more and more. Imagine tension leaving your body with each exhalation.
4.   As you breathe in, slowly count to three. As you breathe out, slowly count to three. Each time you breathe out, repeat a word to yourself—a word such as "peace" or "relax."
5.   Repeat steps 3 and 4 as needed for up to about 20 minutes.
6.   End with a slow deep breath. As you breathe out, say to yourself, "I feel relaxed."

be overcome with thoughtful patient education and reassurances.) Skeptical patients might not construe any benefit to the technique. In some cases, the approach of biofeedback might be more convincing, because the patient receives feedback about biological parameters that improve in response to relaxation techniques.

In a review of nine studies examining the use of R&I alone in pain reduction, only four studies showed a significant difference among pain outcome measures between pretreatment and posttreatment (Carroll and Seers 1998). In only three studies was a significant improvement found when R&I, as compared with a wait-list control condition, was used. This analysis suggests that although R&I can have some efficacy in mitigating pain experiences, it probably is not sufficient as a sole intervention. Compared with alternative treatments, behavior therapy was found to be more effective than R&I, and in another study, biofeedback was found to yield better long-term results than R&I when patients at 6-month follow-up.

Hypnosis

Hypnosis has been recognized as a legitimate form of medical treatment when administered by an appropriately trained therapist. It is a self-induced state brought on by the patient with the assistance of the hypnotist. The mechanism of pain relief brought on by hypnosis is unclear. Questions arise as to whether it is the pain (unpleasant sensations) that is removed or, rather, the reactions to normally painful stimuli. For example, Esdaile, a surgeon in Bengal, India, reported success in using hypnosis for patients in more than 300 operations in the early 1800s. Although there was a report of significant success using hypnosis, it was also reported that many patients were not entirely pain free. For example, some patients "moved and moaned" or awoke in the midst of the operation and "cried out." Afterward, however, they appeared to be amnestic for the surgery and the pain. In other acute pain settings, patients reacted as if they had pain but subsequently could not recall the painful experience (Barber 1963; Orne 1976).

Current conceptualizations view hypnosis as a form of focused attention that is useful in managing acute and chronic pain states, including headache, fibromyalgia, back pain, trigeminal neuralgia, arthritis, phantom limb pain, and cancer pain. Analgesia produced in response to hypnosis was thought to be brought on by modification of attention control systems (i.e., anterior frontal cortex) within the brain. By invoking the techniques summarized in Table 6–7, the patient develops strategies to not attend to painful signals arising from the thalamus and other pain-mediating subcortical brain structures (Crawford et al. 1998).

Analgesia produced through hypnosis is an active process involving the patient's full cooperation. Imaging technology has supported that the process of hypnosis produces signal changes in areas of the brain concerned with sensation and perception (i.e., the sensory cortex and thalamus) and areas of the brain where sensory information is integrated (Raz and Shapiro 2002).

Hypnotic responsiveness varies considerably from person to person but appears to be a stable trait. A number of scales are available to assess responsiveness to hypnosis (Kurtz and Strube 1996). These scales test the patient's ability to respond to a variety of hypnotic suggestions. The most important factor determining response to hypnosis appears to be the patient's imaginative absorption, on which the skillful hypnotist is able to capitalize (Smyser and Baron 1993). Pain reduction is predicted by imaginative absorption.

Because some patients are less susceptible to hypnosis than others, hypnosis might not be a suitable intervention for every patient with complex pain. Hypnosis requires active psychological engagement with the patient in order to be effective; thus, barriers previously mentioned for R&I can likewise interfere with hypnosis.

Table 6–7.   Techniques of hypnosis

Dissociation	The patient is taught to experience another state, place, or time, such as in a vivid daydream, so as to dissociate from the awareness of pain.
Time disorientation	The patient is taught to distort the perception of time (e.g., experiencing a recurrent painful sensation as rapidly passing).
Substitution of sensations	The patient is taught to substitute the unpleasant sensation with another that is more tolerable or less incapacitating. The technique is most effective if the substituted sensation is not entirely pleasant (e.g., substituting a stabbing pain for a pinching pain).
Displacement	The patient is taught to move the painful sensation to another area of the body. For example, if a pain is experienced in the patient's dominant hand, interfering with work, the patient can learn to displace the pain to the small finger of the other hand—and thereby be less adversely affected by the pain.
Reinterpretation	The patient is taught to alter the meaning of the pain to an interpretation that is better tolerated. The pain encountered after a burn, for example, can be reinterpreted as the efforts of the body to restore healing, to channel soothing fluids to bathe and clean up damaged cells.

Vocational Rehabilitation

Patients with pain can experience significant losses, including the loss of work. Beyond the obvious resultant loss of income, and perhaps medical coverage, the loss of work can imply several other losses for the patient depending on the meaning of work for that person. For many persons, work is a source of self-identity, power, influence, and a social network. Loss of work, therefore, can mean the feared loss of control and a feared loss of usefulness.

Psychiatrists can facilitate pursuit of vocational training, which may be helpful in helping the patient transition back to the workplace. If the patient is not returning to his or her prior work, vocational rehabilitation may serve an instructional role, helping the patient develop skills that will be suitable for other kinds of work. Vocational rehabilitation also may be helpful in fostering the patient's independence, autonomy, and self-efficacy and may assist the patient particularly when there is financial need, ineligibility for disability or compensation, and the need for insurance and medical coverage. Vocational rehabilitation can help the patient go beyond the boundaries of his or her illness. Many state agencies provide vocational and educational services for persons with disabilities that can help patients adapt to a work setting. Within such programs, the patient's interests, skills, aptitudes, limitations imposed by physical and psychiatric conditions, and employment needs are assessed. On the basis of these assessments, work training and supervision are provided, with eventual job placement being the ultimate goal.

Key Points

- Effective pain management requires multidimensional approaches. Psychotherapeutic interventions are often necessary for managing pain as well as its psychiatric comorbidities.
- Psychotherapeutic measures can be useful in the comprehensive management of pain to address comorbid psychiatric conditions and subsyndromal psychological states interfering with rehabilitation, and in reducing the adversity produced by the pain itself.
- Psychotherapeutic techniques employed in multidimensional approaches to pain can include the following: supportive therapy, behavior therapy, cognitive-behavioral therapy, dynamic therapy, family/couples therapy, and group therapy.
- In clinical practice, psychotherapists are likely to invoke elements of the varied psychotherapeutic approaches to address the patient's needs.
- Adjuvant approaches, used alone or in combination with psychotherapeutic interventions, include relaxation and imagery training, biofeedback, hypnosis, and vocational rehabilitation.
- Special needs may arise in the palliative care setting, with attention directed to assisting patients with issues arising from existential concerns and spiritual issues.

References

Affleck G, Tennen H, Urrows S, et al: Individual differences in the day-to-day experience of chronic pain: a prospective daily study of rheumatoid arthritis patients. Health Psychol 10:419–426, 1991

Back and Neck Injury/Chronic Pain: Chronic Pain Anonymous. Available at: http://www.backandneck.miningco.com/library/blchair.html. Accessed June 1, 2002.

Barber TX: The effects of "hypnosis" on pain. Psychosom Med 25:303–333, 1963

Beutler LE, Engle D, Oro-Beutler ME, et al: Inability to express intense affect: a common link between depression and pain? J Consult Clin Psychol 54:752–759, 1986

Block A, Kremer E, Gaylor M: Behavioral treatment of chronic pain: the spouse as a discriminative cue for pain behavior. Pain 9:243–252, 1980

Burns JW: Anger management style and hostility: predicting symptom-specific physiological reactivity among chronic low back pain patients. J Behav Med 20:505–522, 1997

Carroll D, Seers K: Relaxation for the relief of chronic pain: a systematic review. J Adv Nurs 27:476–487, 1998

Cogan R, Cogan D, Waltz W, et al: Effects of laughter and relaxation on discomfort thresholds. J Behav Med 10:139–144, 1987

Compas BE, Haaga DAF, Keefe FJ, et al: Sampling of empirically supported psychological treatments from health psychology: smoking, chronic pain, cancer, and bulimia nervosa. J Consult Clin Psychol 66:89–112, 1998

Crawford H, Knebel T, Vendemia JMC: The nature of hypnotic analgesia: neurophysiological foundation and evidence. Contemporary Hypnosis 15:22–34, 1998

Daake DR, Gueldner SH: Imagery instruction and the control of postsurgical pain. Appl Nurs Res 2:114–120, 1989

DeGood DE, Tait RC: Assessment of pain beliefs and pain coping, in Handbook of Pain Assessment, 2nd Edition. Edited by Turk DC, Melzack R. New York, Guilford, 2001, pp 320–345

Feuerstein M: Ambulatory monitoring of paraspinal skeletal muscle, autonomic and mood–pain interaction in chronic low back pain. Paper presented at the 7th annual meeting of the Society of Behavioral Medicine, San Francisco, CA, March 5–8, 1986

Fishman B, Loscalzo M: Cognitive-behavioral interventions in management of cancer pain: principles and applications. Med Clin North Am 71:271–287, 1987

Fordyce WE, Shelton JL, Dundore DE: The modification of avoidance learning pain behaviors. J Behav Med 5:405–414, 1982

Fordyce WE, Roberts AH, Sternbach RA: The behavioral management of chronic pain: a response to critics. Pain 22:113–125, 1985

Hatch JP, Schoenfeld LS, Boutros NN, et al: Anger and hostility in tension-type headache. Headache 31:302–304, 1991

Hawley DJ, Wolfe F: Anxiety and depression in patients with rheumatoid arthritis: a prospective study of 400 patients. J Rheumatol 15:932–941, 1988

Keefe FJ, Dunsmore J, Burnett R: Behavioral and cognitive-behavioral approaches to chronic pain: recent advances and future directions. J Consult Clin Psychol 60:528–536, 1992

Keefe FJ, Baupre PM, Gil KM: Group therapy for patients with chronic pain, in Psychosocial Approaches to Pain Management: A Practitioner's Handbook. Edited by Gatchel RJ, Turk DC. New York, Guilford, 1996, pp 259–282

Kerns RD, Haythornthwaite J: Depression among chronic pain patients: cognitive-behavioral analysis and effects on rehabilitation outcome. J Consult Clin Psychol 56:870–876, 1988

Kerns RD, Turk DC: Depression and chronic pain: the mediating role of the spouse. J Marriage Fam 46:845–852, 1984

Krystal H: Alexithymia and the effectiveness of psychoanalytic treatment. Int J Psychoanal Psychother 9:353–388, 1982

Kurtz RM, Strube MJ: Multiple susceptibility testing: is it helpful? Am J Clin Hypn 38:172–184, 1996

Lakoff R: Interpretive psychotherapy with chronic pain patients. Can J Psychiatry 28:650–653, 1983

Mannix LK, Chandurkar RS, Rybicki LA, et al: Effect of guided imagery on quality of life for patients with chronic tension-type headache. Headache 39:326–334, 1999

McCaffery M, Beebe A: Pain: Clinical Manual for Nursing Practice, 2nd Edition. St Louis, MO, CV Mosby, 1999

Miller WR, Sanchez VC: Motivating young adults for treatment and lifestyle change, in Alcohol Use and Misuse by Young Adults. Edited by Howard G, Nathan PE. Notre Dame, IN, University of Notre Dame Press, 1994, pp 55–82

Morley S, Eccleston C, Williams A: Systematic review and meta-analysis of randomized controlled trials of cognitive behaviour therapy and behaviour therapy for chronic pain in adults, excluding headache. Pain 80:1–13, 1999

Orne MT: Mechanisms of hypnotic pain control, in Advances in Pain Research and Therapy, Vol 1. Edited by Bonica JJ, Albe-Fessard D. New York, Raven, 1976, pp 717–726

Prochaska JO, DiClemente CC: Stages and processes of self-change of smoking: toward an integrative model of change. J Consult Clin Psychol 51:390–395, 1983

Raz A, Shapiro T: Hypnosis and neuroscience: a cross talk between clinical and cognitive research. Arch Gen Psychiatry 59:85–90, 2002

Romano JM, Schmaling KB: Assessment of couples and families with chronic pain, in Handbook of Pain Assessment, 2nd Edition. Edited by Turk DC, Melzack R. New York, Guilford, 2001, pp 346–361

Sanders SH: Operant therapy with pain patients: evidence for its effectiveness, in Seminars in Pain Medicine, Vol 1. Edited by Lebovits AH. Philadelphia, PA, WB Saunders, 2003, pp 90–98

Scheer SJ, Watanabe TK, Radack KL: Randomized controlled trials in industrial low back pain, Part 3: subacute/chronic pain interventions. Arch Phys Med Rehabil 78:414–423, 1997

Seligman MEP: Learned Optimism. New York, Pocket Books, 1990

Sholevar GP, Perkel R: Family systems intervention and physical illness. Gen Hosp Psychiatry 12:363–372, 1990

Silver BV, Blanchard EB: Biofeedback and relaxation training in the treatment of psychophysiological disorders: or are the machines really necessary? J Behav Med 1:217–239, 1978

Smyser CH, Baron DA: Hypnotizability, absorption, and subscales of the Dissociative Experiences Scale in a nonclinical population. Dissociation: Progress in the Dissociative Disorders 6:42–46, 1993

Stieg RL, Lippe P, Shepard TA: Roadblocks to effective pain treatment. Med Clin North Am 83:809–821, 1999

Sullivan MJL, Bishop S, Pivik J: The pain catastrophizing scale: development and validation. Psychol Assess 7:524–532, 1995

Sullivan MJL, Stanish W, Waite H, et al: Catastrophizing, pain, and disability in patients with soft-tissue injuries. Pain 77:253–260, 1998

Tauschke E, Merskey H, Helmes E: Psychological defence mechanisms in patients with pain. Pain 40:161–170, 1990

Turk DC, Meichenbaum DH, Berman WH: Application of biofeedback for the regulation of pain: a critical review. Psychol Bull 86:1322–1338, 1979

Turner JA, Chapman CR: Psychological interventions for chronic pain: a critical review, I: relaxation training and biofeedback. Pain 12:1–21, 1982a

Turner JA, Chapman CR: Psychological interventions for chronic pain: a critical review, II: operant conditioning, hypnosis, and cognitive-behavioral therapy. Pain 12:23–46, 1982b

Weickgenant AL, Slater MA, Patterson TL, et al: Coping activities in chronic low back pain: relationship with depression. Pain 53:95–103, 1993

Weisberg JN, Keefe FJ: Personality, individual differences, and psychopathology in chronic pain, in Psychosocial Factors in Pain. Edited by Gatchel RJ, Turk DC. New York, Guilford, 1999, pp 56–73

7

Special Techniques in
Pain Management

There are a number of therapeutic modalities and interventions available for management of acute and chronic pain (Loeser et al. 2001). The appropriateness of an intervention depends in part on the etiology and nature of the patient's pain, the potential risks of the procedure, and the likelihood of beneficial effects. Generally, conservative modalities are employed first. Certain procedures (e.g., acupuncture, physical therapy) carry relatively fewer risks than more aggressive interventions (e.g., neurosurgical interventions). However, if less invasive measures fail, one may advance in terms of the number of concurrent modalities applied and eventually perhaps to those interventions that carry more risk (see Table 7–1).

It should be noted that highly invasive procedures, although useful, are not a panacea. For example, back pain patients randomly assigned to lumbar fusion surgery or noninvasive educational/exercise programs did not differ significantly at 1-year follow-up on measures of perceived disability, subjective pain ratings, use of analgesics, and general life satisfaction (Brox et al. 2003).

Table 7–1.   Treatment interventions for management of acute and chronic pain conditions

Least invasive	Moderately invasive	Most invasive
Physical therapy	Botox injection	Neurostimulation
Massage	Trigger point injection	Implantable drug pumps
Chiropractic manipulation	Peripheral nerve blocks	Neuroablation/neurolysis
Transcutaneous electrical nerve stimulation	Epidural/intrathecal blocks	Surgical interventions
Acupuncture	Thermal procedures	
Transcranial magnetic stimulation[a]	Prolotherapy	

[a]Preliminary evidence only.

Similarly, comprehensive interdisciplinary treatment programs (largely based on cognitive-behavioral therapy combined with exercise therapy) produced effects that were comparable to those of lumbar spine fusion surgery at 2-year follow-up (Fairbank et al. 2005). Although measures of disability were reduced slightly more among the surgically treated patients, there were no significant differences between the two groups of patients with regard to posttreatment depression or perceived physical and mental health. These data highlight the beneficial impact of psychologically based therapies (see also Chapter 6, "Psychotherapy," of this book) combined with relatively noninvasive procedures in the long-term management of patients with chronic pain. In fact, such rehabilitative endeavors are likely to be more cost-effective than highly invasive (and riskier) interventions (Rivero-Arias et al. 2005).

A brief overview of some of these interventions is presented in this chapter. I also discuss the role of psychiatrists in the care of patients who are pursuing specialized treatment techniques.

Acupuncture

Acupuncture is among the oldest forms of pain intervention, dating as far back as 2600 BCE. Its use has been applied to patients with acute and chronic pain, but the mechanism of action remains unclear. Acupuncture has been a source of marked controversy in Western medicine because of the lack of clear understanding of its physiologic effects. One reason for this lack of understanding is that the points of stimulation in acupuncture are derived from ancient Chinese beliefs about disease processes and are frequently not related to known nervous system pathways.

Nonetheless, anecdotal evidence does support that the technique of acupuncture, if performed properly, can produce significant physiologic changes, some of which have pain-mitigating effects (Brown et al. 1974; Han and Terenius 1982; Mayer et al. 1977). These changes can include increasing endorphin levels within the central nervous system (CNS) (naloxone antagonizes the effectiveness of acupuncture); augmenting other neurotransmitters, including dopamine, serotonin, and norepinephrine (use of serotonin-blocking agents can reduce analgesic effects produced by acupuncture, whereas agents such as clomipramine may possibly augment acupuncture-induced analgesia); alteration of electroencephalographic and cortical evoked potentials; and other potentially beneficial physiologic effects (e.g., vasodilation). Acupuncture has been employed in a number of pain states, including headache, musculoskeletal pains, fibromyalgia, arthritis, bursitis, and synovitis.

Needles (20–100 gauge) are inserted at varying angles through the skin, corresponding to the areas that can mediate pain in various parts of the body. Once the needles are in place, stimulation at the insertion sites is produced by manual manipulation of the needles (e.g., rotated in place, oscillated, or raised up and down with a twirling motion) or through electrical stimulation. Electrical stimulation is less labor intensive and allows for more homogenous and consistent stimulation than manual manipulation techniques.

Fainting, seizures, infection, and pneumothorax (if needles are inserted into the trunk) are some of the potential complications. Needles can break after insertion, requiring surgical excision. When electrical currents are applied to the needle, localized skin burns can result. Patients receiving anticoagulants may be prone to bleeding and hemorrhage. Patients with rheumatic heart disease can develop bacterial endocarditis as a complication of acupuncture. Because of the changes in the vasculature arising from acupuncture, hypovolemic patients might be particularly prone to syncope. Acupuncture has led to spontaneous abortion in the first 3 months of pregnancy and thus should be avoided in the first trimester.

Transcutaneous Electrical Nerve Stimulation

Transcutaneous electrical nerve stimulation (TENS) is a modality employed to reduce pain in an array of acute and chronic pain states, including labor pain, postoperative pain, neuropathic pain, and musculoskeletal pain (Loeser et al. 1975; Tyler et al. 1982). When TENS is used in such settings, patients require less in the way of analgesics (e.g., opiates) and, depending on the circumstances, report increased activity, less interference with work, and improved functional abilities. A TENS unit consists of a battery and electrodes. The electrodes are placed along the surface of the skin overlying painful areas. The battery generates electrical currents of approximately 100 milliamperes; the rate and width of the pulses are modifiable by the patient. The efficacy of TENS has been supported by evidence of counterirritation techniques (see also Chapter 2, "Sensory Pathways of Pain and Acute Versus Chronic Pain," of this book), whereby stimulation of $A\beta$ fibers inhibits the pain-promoting activities within the substantia gelatinosa.

Prolotherapy

Prolotherapy is a long-described intervention whereby pain of musculoskeletal origin is treated by injection of a dextrose/lidocaine solution into connective tissue sites that are thought to be related to the genesis and perpetuation of pain. Prolotherapy has been used in the treatment of discogenic low back pain; chronic cervical, thoracic, or lumbar pain; osteoarthritis; and failed back surgery (postspinal surgery) pain (Linetsky et al. 2006). Contraindications include treatment of patients with pain related to neoplastic processes and patients requiring large quantities of narcotic analgesics before and after treatment. Prolotherapy may be employed in conjunction with other procedures (e.g., peripheral nerve blocks).

Botulinum Toxin (Botox) Injection

The neurotoxins produced by *Clostridium botulinum* exert physiologic effects by inhibiting release of acetylcholine from nerve terminals. These effects account for the utility of botulinum injections in alleviating blepharospasm or facial spasm but not necessarily pain. Analgesic effects of botulinum toxin type A may involve other neurotransmitter influences, including inhibition of glutamate and substance P. Botulinum toxin (both A and B types) has been invoked in the treatment of cervical dystonia, migraine headache, tension headache, temporomandibular joint disorders, and chronic back pain (Argoff 2005). Multiple series of injections may be required to achieve maximal analgesia. Contraindications include pregnancy, concurrent aminoglycoside antibiotic use (e.g., gentamicin, tobramycin), myasthenia gravis, Eaton-Lambert syndrome, and known sensitivity to toxins. Clinical resistance brought on by development of antibodies to toxins may reduce clinical efficacy after repeated administrations.

Anesthesia at the Level of the Spinal Cord

Anesthesia at the level of the spinal cord involves application of anesthetics to influence spinal or sympathetic nerves, or both, to produce pain relief. Epidural anesthesia involves application of the anesthetic outside the dura mater—the dura mater is not punctured (at least not intentionally). Epidural anesthesia has become the cornerstone of acute pain management (e.g., operative and postoperative pain). Intrathecal (subarachnoid) application of anesthetics involves inserting a needle through the dura mater and applying the anesthetic into the cerebrospinal fluid. Both epidural and intrathecal analgesia are invoked in the management of patients with chronic pain in whom pharmacologic interventions produce intolerable side effects or are insufficient to control pain.

The subarachnoid administration of anesthetics allows for more direct access of anesthetics to pain-relaying and sympathetic nerves. On the other hand, the epidural space contains areolar (fat) tissue, epidural veins, and lymphatic tissue, into which the anesthetic will diffuse and be absorbed. Thus, epidural administration is an indirect means of providing blockade of pain-sensitive nerves entering the spinal cord. Because of the distance traveled by the anesthetic agent and absorption of the agent by the fat layer surrounding the dura, anesthetics introduced in this manner take a longer time to exert a full effect. In addition, less intense sensory (and motor) blockade results from epidural injection compared with subarachnoid injection. Consequently, in achieving anesthesia through the epidural technique, generally more anesthetic is required than is the case for subarachnoid injections. The dura mater is not penetrated or broken through, so post–spinal-injection headache and meningitis are less likely to occur with epidural injection. Epidural anesthesia is also less likely to produce cardiovascular effects that are observed with subarachnoid injections.

Neural influences occur in a sequential manner after the anesthetic is introduced. Because fibers are small and unmyelinated and are more susceptible to the effects of the anesthetic agents than are the larger myelinated fibers, sympathetic nerves are blocked first. This is followed by involvement of sensory fibers and subsequently motor nerves. Motor fibers tend to be deeper in the nerves, and, thus, greater diffusion of the anesthetic is required to influence motor blockade.

Complications associated with subarachnoid and epidural injections are summarized in Table 7–2. Puncture of the dura mater during an intended epidural injection, referred to as "wet tap," can produce significant headache. After subarachnoid injection, analgesia and paralysis may be produced at levels higher than intended (i.e., high spinal). In this way, sympathetic innervation to vital organs arising from thoracic spinal segments can be inadvertently suppressed, resulting in compromised cardiac output and ventilatory mechanics. Contraindications for both techniques are also outlined in Table 7–2 (Barash et al. 2001).

Multiple agents can be administered via the subarachnoid and epidural techniques, including opiates, steroids, α_2-adrenergic agonists (e.g., clonidine), and muscle relaxants (e.g., baclofen). Continuous opiate analgesia may be applied through implantable drug delivery systems inserted through the epidural or subarachnoid route. These systems are often employed in patients with cancer pain and are being increasingly explored in chronic, nonmalignant pain. Risks associated with continuous implantable infusions are summarized in Table 7–3.

Regional Neural Blockade

Regional neural blockade (RNB) encompasses a number of techniques whereby nociceptive inputs of nerve fibers are interrupted (e.g., peripheral or sympathetic nerve blockade). The purpose of RNB is multifaceted. RNB can serve a diagnostic function, helping to decipher peripheral nerve pain from sympathetically mediated pain. Some procedures may be invoked to provide prophylaxis of future pain after surgical procedures (e.g., to minimize phantom limb pain postamputation). In addition, RNB techniques may be invoked to provide therapeutic pain relief in selected disorders, especially in those chronic pain disorders involving sympathetically mediated pain and complex regional

Table 7–2.   Complications and contraindications of subarachnoid and epidural analgesia

Complications	Contraindications
Subarachnoid	**Absolute**
Hypotension	Lack of patient consent
Post–spinal-injection headache	Allergy or sensitivities to local anesthetics
High spinal[a]	Increased intracranial pressure
Nausea, vomiting	Infection at the potential puncture site
Urinary retention	**Relative**
Backache	Hypovolemia
Epidural	Coagulopathy
Unintentional injection of anesthetic	Sepsis
Into subarachnoid space	Progressive neurologic diseases
Into vascular space	Chronic back pain
"Wet tap"	
Local anesthetic overdose	
Hypotension	
Spinal cord trauma	
Epidural hematoma	

[a]Analgesia and paralysis produced at levels higher than intended.

pain syndrome. At times, RNB is employed to determine the suitability of other more permanent interventions (e.g., neural destruction techniques). The types of RNB techniques and the ways in which these are employed, as well as complications and indications, have been summarized extensively elsewhere (Barash et al. 2001).

Table 7–3.   Risks of continuous epidural or subarachnoid anesthetic infusions

Catheter problems
   Moving
   Kinking
   Breaking
   Disconnection
   Occlusion (by fibrosis in epidural placement site)
Infection
   Local infection
   Epidural abscess
   Meningitis

Peripheral Nerve Blockade

When pain is refractory to pharmacologic treatment, peripheral nerve blockade may be an option (Raj 1996). Somatic nerve blocks are used in patients with intractable pain, generally from cancerous invasion of parts of the body, including the nervous system. At times, these blocks are employed in peripheral nerve pain, sciatica, and carpal tunnel syndrome. In addition, peripheral nerve blocks are employed to provide analgesia during localized surgery so that the patient can avoid general anesthesia.

Nerve blocks can include anesthetic and ablative modalities (see Table 7–4). In the case of anesthetic blockade, introduction of local anesthetics (lidocaine or bupivacaine) allows for interruption of pain transmission, producing effective, albeit temporary, pain relief. The activity of thin and unmyelinated nerve fibers (e.g., Aδ and C fibers) is particularly prone to inhibition, requiring minimal doses of anesthetic agents. If higher doses are used, it is possible to inhibit larger myelinated fibers, such as motor neurons. Pain interruption might be of sufficient duration to allow the patient to become more proactive with physical therapy, which in turn might set the stage for further health improvements and rehabilitation. Ablative techniques involve application of ethanol or phenol or other interventions (see Table 7–4) that result in permanent destruction of the nerve. Neural destruction is never attempted unless local application of anesthetics has first been tried. If local anesthetics fail to produce pain relief, it is unlikely that neural destruction will be effective in mitigating pain.

Anesthetic infusions can produce untoward effects (e.g., hypotension, localized numbness, muscle weakness, infection, bleeding). Such measures should never be attempted unless resuscitation equipment is readily available.

Sympathetic Nerve Blockade

As with peripheral nerve blockade, a number of comparable measures may be undertaken to reduce pain that is sympathetically mediated. Complex pain syndromes involving the arm, head, and neck might benefit from a stellate ganglion block. Similarly, diffuse pain in the lower extremities can benefit from a lumbar sympathetic block. Visceral pain syndromes (e.g., pain arising from the pancreas and other upper abdominal organs) can be mitigated by celiac plexus block; pain originating from pelvic organs can be reduced with hypogastric plexus block (Eisenberg et al. 1995). Such measures may not provide

Table 7–4. Modalities of regional nerve blockade

Type of intervention	Purpose	Examples
Anesthetic blockade	Use of local anesthetics to interrupt nociceptive input from peripheral nerves	Interscalene, supraclavicular and infraclavicular, axillary, sciatic nerve, and lumbar plexus blocks
Neuroablative blockade	Use of chemical, thermal, cryogenic, or surgical modalities applied to induce intentional nerve injury to reduce pain transmission from the periphery; often impermanent, lasting 3–6 months	Peripheral nerve ablation for focal pain related to cancer invasion; sympathetic nerve ablation for visceral, retroperitoneal, and complex regional pain syndrome related to cancer

Table 7–5.   Types of and uses for autonomic nerve blocks

Type of nerve block	Uses

Celiac plexus block	Pain arising from viscera, secondary to cancer
	    Pancreas
	    Alimentary tract (esophagus through transverse
	        colon)

Hypogastric plexus block	Pelvic, vaginal, scrotal pain Buttock, inguinal pain
Lumbar sympathetic block	Complex regional pain syndrome Neuropathic pain (e.g., postherpetic neuralgia) Vascular insufficiency
Sphenopalatine ganglion block	Frontal headache Cluster headache Migraine headache
Stellate ganglion block	Complex regional pain syndrome Postherpetic neuralgia Intractable angina pectoris Vascular insufficiency (e.g., Raynaud disease, scleroderma)

Superior mesenteric
    ganglion block
	Pain arising from viscera, secondary to cancer
	    Bladder, kidney, ureters
	    Distal colon, rectum
	    Prostate, testicle
	    Uterus

complete pain relief. However, even if only partial relief is achieved, this may be sufficient to allow the patient to lower the amount of opiate analgesics required, thereby reducing the risks of untoward effects.

Sympathetic nerve blockades are employed in conditions of unremitting pain arising from the viscera, generally induced by cancer. In some cases, the use of opiate analgesics and adjuvants proves to be unsatisfactory or intolerable. Types of and uses for autonomic nerve blocks are summarized in Table 7–5.

Neurosurgical Techniques

Neurosurgical techniques consist of anatomic, augmentative (i.e., neural stimulation), and ablative techniques (see Table 7–6). Anatomic interventions are relatively common interventions that correct defects (e.g., disc herniations)

Table 7–6. Neurosurgical interventions for use in pain management

Type of intervention	Purpose	Examples
Anatomic	Reduce compression of nerve fibers; reduce pain and improve neurologic effects	Laminectomy Discectomy Microvascular decompression
Augmentative	Stimulate the neural axis to reduce pain; can be costly but is relatively safe and reversible	Spinal nerve stimulation Peripheral nerve stimulation Intracranial stimulation
Ablative	Generally, interventions of last resort, predominantly patients with terminal conditions	
Peripheral	Denervate an area of the body	Sympathectomy Neurectomy Ganglionectomies Rhizotomy of cranial nerves
Spinal	Destroy pain input; relief is often time limited; there can be neurologic complications	Dorsal root entry zone lesioning Cordotomy Myelotomy
Brain	Disrupt widespread pain transmission intracranially; effects are often short-term	Thalamotomy Cingulotomy

that produce neurologic deficits and pain. Presumably, correction of the anatomic defect will reduce pain and restore neurologic functioning (e.g., weakness due to nerve impingement).

Augmentative, or stimulation, techniques are employed to suppress the activity of nerves relaying painful information. Inhibition is rather dramatic, such that when high-frequency, low-amplitude stimulation is applied, dorsal horn cell activity is inhibited (Meyerson and Linderoth 2001). Stimulation techniques have been used in chronic, intractable pain affecting the limbs or the trunk, including conditions such as phantom limb pain, arachnoiditis, neuropathy, and complex regional pain syndrome.

Neural stimulation techniques may be employed within the CNS (i.e., through implantable devices inserted within the spinal column to stimulate the dorsal horn) or peripherally. The peripheral technique is employed to treat neurogenic pain in the limbs; a generator and stimulation electrodes are placed beneath the skin, and the electrodes are placed in proximity to the peripheral nerve.

Because spinal cord stimulation is such a complex procedure, this approach is reserved for those patients whose pain has been refractory to other interventions or for whom other interventions prove intolerable. Stimulation is not allowable in patients who have a demand cardiac pacemaker, who require magnetic resonance imaging in the immediate future, or who have ongoing substance dependence. In addition, because of the invasiveness of this procedure, there must be a clearly identified basis for the nature of the pain.

In general, ablative techniques are invoked for severe, refractory pain conditions, particularly in patients with cancer-related pain. Ablative techniques involve removal or destruction of nerve centers or other components of pain pathways, at the level of peripheral or cranial nerves (e.g., trigeminal ganglion ablation), spinal cord, or brain.

Repetitive Transcranial Magnetic Stimulation

An emerging therapy, transcranial magnetic stimulation (TMS), has been demonstrated to be useful in treating a number of conditions involving disturbances in neural circuitry (i.e., depression, seizures, and other neurologic conditions). TMS is a technology whereby an electrical current is passed through an insulated circular or figure-eight coil to produce a magnetic pulse. When the coil is applied to the head, the magnetic pulse is capable of passing uninterrupted through the skin and skull, and ultimately to the cortex. When a series of pulses repeated at equal intervals are generated, referred to as repetitive TMS (rTMS), it is possible to modify neuronal activity locally in focal regions of the cortex and at distant (i.e., subcortical) sites (Wassermann and Lisanby 2001).

Literature has emerged that suggests that TMS may have potential utility in treating neuropathic pain. In a review of studies assessing the influence of rTMS in neuropathic pain, it was noted that rTMS was able to produce pain relief but often analgesia was brief (Leo and Latif 2007). The influence of rTMS appears to be best when high-frequency stimulation is applied and when the site of stimulation is focused over the motor cortex (as compared with other cortical sites).

rTMS is a noninvasive strategy with a benign side-effect profile; it is easy to administer. Although adverse effects are minimal, its practical application and efficacy for pain treatment have yet to be determined by further empirical investigation.

Role of the Psychiatrist in Pain Management Related to Interventions

There are several aspects to the psychiatrist's role in the care of patients undergoing any of the aforementioned interventions. By spanning preintervention to postintervention (see Table 7–7), the psychiatrist can be helpful in ensuring that the patient is prepared for the intervention and continues to participate in functional restoration measures postintervention.

Table 7–7.   Role of psychiatrists in the care of patients undergoing interventional pain management

Preintervention role	Assess capacity to give informed consent.
	Assist patients in
	Acquiring information necessary to make informed decision regarding interventions.
	Developing realistic expectations of likely outcomes derived from varied interventions.
	Screen patients for conditions
	That preclude undergoing interventions, particularly those that are highly invasive and/or risky.
	That may interfere with yielding optimal benefits from interventions.
	Provide treatment to remediate psychiatric comorbidities that may (if untreated) preclude, or limit efficacy of, interventions.
Postintervention role	Facilitate patient participation in other facets of the rehabilitation process.
	Assist patients with managing pain, activity limitations, disappointments arising after an intervention is pursued.

Preintervention Role

Psychiatrists may be enlisted to assess the mental and cognitive abilities of the patient to give consent to undergo a procedure, particularly if the procedure is highly invasive. Unlike *competency,* which requires a judicial determination as to the person's possession of the requisite natural or legal qualifications to engage in an endeavor, *capacity* is determined by the physician (often, although not exclusively, by a psychiatrist). A capacity assessment essentially determines the validity of a patient's decision to undergo or forgo a particular proposed treatment. Table 7–8 summarizes a reasonable guide for the physician assessing a patient's decision-making capacity (Leo 1999). With highly invasive procedures, one must carefully weigh the risks of the proposed procedure against the potential benefits. The psychiatrist must ensure that the patient has sufficient cognitive and psychological skills to understand the illness, the proposed intervention, its risks and benefits, and the likely long-term outcomes of a procedure. Inquiries should be directed to the patient, according to the guidelines, and the patient's responses should be systematically recorded in the medical record, preferably as quotations. Failure of the patient to understand, appreciate, and form rational decisions would suggest that the patient does not have the capacity to make reasoned decisions regarding the proposed medical treatment.

If a person lacks the capacity to make treatment decisions, it may be incumbent on the consulting psychiatrist to remedy barriers to capacity. In some cases, disturbances in the doctor–patient relationship (i.e., ineffective communication) might be the sole basis for the lack of capacity. The psychiatrist may be enlisted to clarify and rectify such communication difficulties. In other cases, a psychiatric disturbance (e.g., delirium, psychosis, a mood disorder) may be impeding the patient's capacity to give informed consent, but once the condition is rectified (e.g., through use of medication, therapy) the patient is able to do so.

If the patient lacks capacity and the problem is not remediable, the treating clinician (other than a psychiatrist) may need to invoke substituted consent. Although states vary as to who may be appointed as a substitute, this role often falls to spouses, relatives, ethics boards, and so forth. In some situations, a judicial decision of incompetence is required. If so deemed, the patient would have a court-appointed guardian assigned to make medical decisions on his or her behalf.

Despite possession of a knowledge base suggesting that they possess requisite skills to make decisions, some patients may, nonetheless, harbor overly optimistic and unrealistic expectations of the outcome of an intervention. In

Table 7–8.   Psychiatrists' guide for assessing patient decision-making capacity

The patient must demonstrate an understanding of each of the following:

1. Current medical condition
2. Natural course of his or her current medical condition
3. Proposed treatment intervention
4. Potential risks and benefits of the proposed treatment intervention
5. Consequences of refusing the proposed treatment intervention
6. Presence of any viable alternatives to the proposed treatment intervention
7. Potential risks and benefits of alternative treatments

Source.   Adapted from Leo RJ: "Competency and the Capacity to Make Treatment Decisions: A Primer for Primary Care Physicians." *Primary Care Companion to the Journal of Clinical Psychiatry* 1:131–141, 1999. Copyright 1999, Physicians Postgraduate Press. Used with permission.

reality, there are no guarantees of the success of interventions undertaken on behalf of the patient with chronic pain. Sometimes, patients present with permanent, irreversible damage, such that the pain will not be resolved entirely no matter how effective the intervention is purported to be. It may be prudent, therefore, for psychiatrists to work with the patient in establishing realistic expectations regarding selected interventions and treatment goals. It may become necessary to ascertain the patient's preparedness for the risks or untoward effects potentially associated with an intervention.

Psychiatrists may be enlisted to assess the patient's suitability for various interventions (e.g., identifying whether psychiatric conditions would interfere with outcome) (Trief et al. 2000). The extent of involvement of a psychiatrist in determining patient suitability depends in part on the severity/aggressiveness of the intervention. The least invasive procedures may not warrant psychiatric prescreening, whereas more invasive procedures (e.g., neurosurgical interventions) would warrant such evaluation (Nelson et al. 1996). The presence of major psychiatric disturbances (e.g., psychosis, major mood disorders, somatoform disorders, suicidality) is likely to predict poor response to surgical interventions. Patients with ambiguous conditions (i.e., inconsistent physical findings, poorly defined pain, or pain without neurologic correlates) are not likely to have successful results with highly invasive interventions (Block et al. 2003). Significant cognitive deficits contraindicate such interventions as well, because the cognitively impaired patient is not likely to adhere to treatment and may lack the wherewithal to mobilize medical assistance if complications arise. Similarly, refractory substance abuse, deception, and threats to treating sources that drastic measures will be undertaken if the interventions are not undertaken may preclude pursuit of invasive interventions (see also the section "Evaluation of Treatment Suitability" in Chapter 3, "Evaluation of the Pain Patient," of this book).

Other factors that may raise concerns about patient suitability for various interventions may include a history of treatment nonadherence, use of large amounts of narcotics and/or anxiolytics (raising concerns regarding substance dependence), and concerns over behaviors suggesting secondary gain (e.g., ongoing litigation issues) (Block et al. 2003). Careful consideration of such factors might warrant that invasive procedures be delayed until corrective measures can be put in place (e.g., treatment of comorbid depression or substance dependence). Similarly, psychiatrists may be instrumental in eliciting patient adherence with other related facets to the patient's treatment. It may be particularly helpful to engage the patient in weight reduction measures, smoking cessation, participation in exercise programs, and relaxation training, before attempts are made at intervening with more aggressive interventions. When undertaken, such endeavors convey that the patient is taking on a proactive role in his or her rehabilitation. Patient refusal with such measures may be an indication that aggressive interventions may need to be delayed or perhaps withheld altogether.

Postintervention Role

It may become necessary to assist patients who are disappointed over unachieved outcomes, or less than optimal results, after an intervention has been undertaken. Pain relief may be only partial, and there may be residual physical activity limitations that persist after an intervention, necessitating psychiatric follow-up. Strong reactions such as alarm ("Something has gone wrong!"), disappointment ("I was hoping I would be better."), and futility ("Nothing will help.") may undermine rehabilitative treatment measures and any potentially achievable gains. Adjunctive treatment modalities such as hypnosis, relaxation and imagery, guided imagery, and biofeedback may be helpful in mitigating pain perception and distress in such cases (see also Chapter 6 in this book). Psychotherapeutic measures may be helpful in assisting patients with reframing such reactions to mitigate any potential undermining of rehabilitative endeavors. Ongoing collaborative endeavors between the psychiatrist and physical and occupational therapists, along with other treating sources, may be essential to assist the patient in overcoming psychological barriers that may impede functional restoration measures postintervention.

Key Points

- Several interventions are available for management of acute and chronic pain, ranging from those that carry few risks to those that are more risky and invasive.

- Interventions warranting consideration for pain management include acupuncture, transcutaneous electrical nerve stimulation, prolotherapy, botulinum toxin injection, epidural and spinal analgesia, nerve blocks, and neurosurgical techniques.

- Patient selection for various interventions is pivotal in achieving efficacy and positive outcomes. Most chronic pain patients respond best when such procedures are part of multidisciplinary treatment approaches encompassing physical therapy, psychotherapy, and vocational rehabilitation.

- Psychiatrists may be involved in assessing the patient's capacity to provide informed consent for and his or her suitability to undergo interventions (particularly those that are highly invasive). It may also be necessary to assist patients in developing realistic expectations regarding likely treatment goals and outcomes.

- Psychiatrists may be enlisted postintervention to assist patients with overcoming psychological barriers that may impede rehabilitative measures.

References

Argoff CE: Botulinum toxin injections, in Pain Medicine and Management: Just the Facts. Edited by Wallace MS, Staats PS. New York, McGraw-Hill, 2005, pp 266–272

Barash PG, Cullen BF, Stoelting RK (eds): Clinical Anesthesia, 4th Edition. Philadelphia, PA, Lippincott Williams & Wilkins, 2001

Block AR, Gatchel RJ, Deardorff WW, et al: The Psychology of Spine Surgery, 1st Edition. Washington, DC, American Psychological Association, 2003

Brown ML, Ulett GA, Stern JA: Acupuncture loci: techniques for location. Am J Chin Med (Gard City N Y) 2:67–74, 1974

Brox JI, Sorenson R, Friis PT, et al: Randomized clinical trial of lumbar instrumental fusion and cognitive intervention and exercises in patients with chronic low back pain and disc degeneration. Spine 28:1913–1921, 2003

Eisenberg E, Carr DB, Chalmers TC: Neurolytic celiac plexus block for treatment of cancer pain: a meta-analysis. Anesth Analg 80:290–295, 1995

Fairbank J, Frost H, Wilson-MacDonald J, et al: Randomised controlled trial to compare surgical stabilisation of the lumbar spine with an intensive rehabilitation programme for patients with chronic low back pain: the MRC spine stabilization trial. BMJ 330:1233–1238, 2005

Han JS, Terenius L: Neurochemical basis of acupuncture analgesia. Annu Rev Pharmacol Toxicol 22:193–220, 1982

Leo RJ: Competency and the capacity to make treatment decisions: a primer for primary care physicians. Prim Care Companion J Clin Psychiatry 1:131–141, 1999

Leo RJ, Latif T: Repetitive transcranial magnetic stimulation (rTMS) in acute and chronic neuropathic pain: a review. J Pain 8:453–459, 2007

Linetsky FS, Derby R, Miguel R, et al: Pain management with regenerative injection therapy, in Weiner's Pain Management: A Practical Guide for Clinicians, 7th Edition. Edited by Boswell MV, Cole BE. Boca Raton, FL, Taylor & Francis Group, 2006, pp 939–965

Loeser JD, Black RG, Christman A: Relief of pain by transcutaneous stimulation. J Neurosurg 42:308–314, 1975

Loeser JD, Butler SH, Chapman CR, et al (eds): Bonica's Management of Pain, 3rd Edition. Philadelphia, PA, Lippincott Williams & Wilkins, 2001

Mayer DJ, Price DD, Rafii A: Antagonism of acupuncture analgesia in man by the narcotic antagonist naloxone. Brain Res 121:368–372, 1977

Meyerson BA, Linderoth B: Spinal cord stimulation, in Bonica's Management of Pain, 3rd Edition. Edited by Loeser JD, Butler SH, Chapman CR, et al. Philadelphia, PA, Lippincott Williams & Wilkins, 2001, pp 1857–1876

Nelson DV, Kennington M, Novy DM, et al: Psychological selection criteria for implantable spinal cord stimulators. Pain Forum 5:93–103, 1996

Raj PP: Peripheral nerve blocks, in Pain Management: A Comprehensive Review. Edited by Raj PP. St Louis, MO, Mosby, 1996, pp 200–226

Rivero-Arias O, Campbell H, Gray A, et al: Surgical stabilization of the spine compared with a programme of intensive rehabilitation for the management of patients with chronic low back pain: cost utility analysis based on a randomized controlled trial. BMJ 330:1239–1243, 2005

Trief PM, Grant W, Fredrickson B: A prospective study of psychological predictors of lumbar surgery outcome. Spine 25:2616–2621, 2000

Tyler E, Caldwell C, Ghia JN: Transcutaneous electrical nerve stimulation: an alternative approach to the management of postoperative pain. Anesth Analg 61:449–456, 1982

Wassermann EM, Lisanby SH: Therapeutic application of repetitive transcranial magnetic stimulation: a review. Clin Neurophysiol 112:1367–1377, 2001

8

Common Pain Disorders

Headache

Headache is among the most prevalent of pain conditions, estimated to account for 10 million office visits annually in the United States (Collins 1986). It is the most common reason for lost worker productivity (Stewart et al. 2003). Evaluation of the patient with headache, and development of treatment strategies, relie primarily on the history, supplemented by physical examination and judicious use of diagnostic testing when indicated by history and physical findings (see Table 8–1). Three common benign headache conditions are discussed briefly below.

Tension Headache

Tension headache is very common, affecting as many as 70% of men and 85% of women annually. Tension headache can also occur among persons with migraine headache—often confounding diagnostic features—but is not any more prevalent among persons with migraine headache. Classically, the features of tension headache involve a pressing and tightening quality that is bilateral and often described as bandlike or surrounding the head (Welch 2001). The in-

Table 8–1.   Evaluation of the headache patient

History	
Characteristic features	Onset
	Temporal patterns
	Duration
	Quality of pain
	Location
	Change in course of one's customary headache
	Associated features
	Aggravating factors
	Mitigating factors
Factors suggesting secondary headache	Environmental factors
	Head trauma/posttrauma
	Infection
	Postlumbar puncture
	Prior pattern of analgesic use (e.g., medication overuse and rebound)
Worrisome symptoms/ features	Fever
	Weight loss
	Altered consciousness
	Stiff neck
	Weakness, gait disturbance
	Abrupt, "split-second" onset
	Onset after age 50 years
	Other conditions (e.g., HIV, cancer)
Physical examination	Blood pressure
	Fundoscopic examination
	Temporal artery tenderness
	Kernig's/Brudzinski's sign
	Neurologic examination
Diagnostic testing	Sedimentation rate
	Head computed tomography with/without contrast
	Head magnetic resonance imaging
	Lumbar puncture
	Magnetic resonance venogram (e.g., suspected sagittal sinus thrombosis)

tensity of tension headache can vary from mild to moderate in severity. Although tension headache can inhibit activities, it does not prohibit them. Tension headache is rarely aggravated by routine activities such as walking and climbing stairs. Generally, tension headache is not accompanied by nausea, vomiting, or photophobia or phonophobia.

Tension headache is thought to arise from peripheral changes (i.e., myofascial pain sensitivity and increased pericranial muscle activity). It can be brought on by physical and psychological stress as well as poor posture and ergonomic conditions. Emotional factors can contribute to the frequency and severity of headache. It is speculated that limbic system activity invoked during emotional distress might both contribute to muscle contraction and inhibit endogenous antinociceptive pathways; however, the exact process remains unclear (Holm et al. 1986).

Treatment of acute episodes of tension headache includes use of nonsteroidal anti-inflammatory drugs (NSAIDs) such as ibuprofen, ketorolac, ketoprofen, and naproxen (see Table 8–2). There does not appear to be any indication for muscle relaxants or analgesics containing opiates. Prophylaxis of tension headache is probably facilitated most by tricyclic antidepressants (TCAs). A TCA can be used for 4 months. If the frequency of headache is reduced significantly, the TCA can be tapered and discontinued. There might be a need to reinstate the TCA for longer-term use if the headaches recur.

In a recent study, nefazodone was effective in treating patients with chronic daily headache. However, patients with comorbid depression had better results from nefazodone than did those who were not depressed (Saper et al. 2001). Other researchers have reported that patients with chronic daily headache had reduced symptoms with amitriptyline, nortriptyline, or stress management. No information was provided about which patients with headache were more apt to benefit from these measures (Holroyd et al. 2001). Serotonin-selective antidepressants, mirtazapine, and venlafaxine might also be efficacious in chronic headache (Ansari 2000; Bendtsen and Jensen 2004; Diamond 1995).

Effective psychotherapeutic modalities include biofeedback training and relaxation training (see Chapter 6, "Psychotherapy," of this book). Stress management therapy and cognitive-behavioral therapy (CBT) may also be helpful in reducing stress levels, but they are probably most effective when combined with relaxation or biofeedback training (Holroyd et al. 1977). Characteristics of patients who are likely to improve with the use of psychotherapeutic treat-

Table 8–2. Treatment of headache

Abortive	Prophylactic
Tension headache	
NSAIDs	Antidepressants
Acetaminophen	Tricyclic antidepressants
Aspirin	SSRIs (e.g., fluoxetine)
	Mirtazapine
	Nefazodone
Migraine headache	
Triptans (e.g., sumatriptan, zolmitriptan, naratriptan)	β-Blockers (e.g., propranolol, timolol)
	Calcium channel blockers (e.g., verapamil)
Ergotamines	Methysergide
NSAIDs	Ergotamines
Butorphanol	Tricyclic antidepressants
Opiates	Anticonvulsants (e.g., divalproex, gabapentin,
Caffeine	topiramate)
Antiemetics	Clonidine
	Botulinum toxin injection
Cluster headache	
Oxygen inhalation	Lithium
Ergotamines	Divalproex sodium/topiramate
Triptans	Calcium channel blockers (e.g., verapamil)
	Ergotamines
	Methysergide
	Steroids

Note.　NSAID = nonsteroidal anti-inflammatory drug; SSRI = selective serotonin reuptake inhibitor.

ment are summarized in Table 8–3. Of these factors, the most striking is that those patients in relaxation training who show positive responses by the fourth session (as measured by muscle level reactivity on electromyogram [EMG]) are likely to have an excellent response to relaxation or biofeedback training (Bogaards and ter Kuile 1994). Uncontrolled studies have revealed that dental complications may predispose some persons to tension headache, and these persons may

Table 8–3. Factors influencing likelihood of response to psychotherapeutic measures in patients with tension headache

Young age of patient

Shorter duration of headache, compared with chronic headache

Relaxation training that produces at least 50% reduction of activity as shown on EMG by the fourth session (predictive of an excellent response)

Lower scores on psychometric measures of depression

Patient's requiring minimal analgesia

Note. EMG=electromyogram.

respond favorably to occlusal adjustments and splints and therapeutic masticatory exercises. Patients with chronic daily headache are often unable to obtain much benefit from psychotherapy interventions. For such patients, the combination of psychotherapy (e.g., CBT) and the judicious use of pharmacologic interventions is likely to yield better clinical improvements than those achieved with either treatment alone (Lake 2001; Lipchik and Nash 2002).

Migraine Headache

Migraine headache occurs less frequently than tension headache, affecting approximately 6% of men and 15%–18% of women. Hormonal influences might account for these gender differences, because the rates of migraine among prepubescent boys and girls are equal (Silberstein 1992). Classically, migraine headache can last approximately 4–72 hours. Generally, these headaches are unilateral, with a pulsating quality. The intensity of migraine headache is moderate to severe (i.e., inhibits and prohibits activities). Migraine headache is often aggravated by routine activities (e.g., walking, climbing stairs). It is often accompanied by photophobia or phonophobia, nausea, and vomiting (Welch 2001).

Migraine headache can be preceded by an aura. Migraine headache without aura is approximately twice as frequent as that with aura. However, both can occur in the same patient. The variability in the features of migraine headache, even in the same person among different episodes, can complicate the diagnosis. Aura precedes migraine headache and develops gradually over several minutes; it is a transient neurologic symptom and generally does not last beyond 60 minutes. The aura is followed by the headache, generally within 60 minutes. At times, migraine headache can be preceded by more than one aura, occur-

Table 8–4.   Common auras associated with migraine headache

Visual
    Flashing lights
    Fortification spectra
    Scotomata
    Hemianopsia
    Visual hallucinations
Auditory
    Abnormal auditory sensations (e.g., tinnitus)
    Auditory hallucinations
    Decreased hearing
Olfactory
    Abnormal olfactory sensations
    Olfactory hallucinations
Sensory
    Paresthesia
    Vertigo
Motor
    Weakness

ring in succession. Auras must be distinguished from other neurologic symptoms that can signal other disorders (e.g., seizure, transient ischemic attacks). The commonly encountered auras are listed in Table 8–4. Given that these symptoms can mimic symptoms of other disorders and can trigger marked patient and physician distress, psychiatric evaluation of the patient might be requested. Careful assessment of the patient is warranted to differentiate symptoms of migraine (e.g., visual or auditory hallucinations) from those of psychiatric disorders such as schizophrenia or delirium. Differentiating these features from functional psychiatric disorders is possible by referring to the patient's longitudinal history, family history, and presence of cognitive and other neurologic symptoms. The transience of auras and their temporal relationship to headache and other migraine features suggest migraine headache instead of functional psychiatric disorders. The clinician is cautioned against hastily initiating antipsychotic medications and thus failing to appropriately evaluate and treat the migraine condition. Of most concern is that other serious conditions (e.g., transient ischemic attacks) may be dismissed as reflecting functional psychiatric disturbances, and workup and appropriate treatment (e.g., with clopidogrel) might be overlooked.

Common precipitants of migraine headache include alcohol use, emotional distress, and menstruation. It is interesting to note that migraine headache frequency appears to decline during pregnancy and menopause, supporting the notion that hormonal factors have an impact on migraine headache. However, hormone therapy during menopause can prolong the migraine condition even after menopause (Epstein et al. 1975). Certain psychiatric disorders (e.g., childhood somnambulism) may possibly predict adulthood migraine headache. Other common psychiatric comorbidities among migraineurs include depression, anxiety disorders (e.g., generalized anxiety and panic disorder), and bipolar disorder (particularly bipolar II disorder) (Breslau et al. 2003; Fasmer 2001; Zwart et al. 2003).

Treatment of migraine headache depends on the frequency and severity of the headaches, the presence of neurologic symptoms, and the impact of potential interventions on the patient's lifestyle. Headaches occurring once per month or less might require only abortive therapies, whereas those of greater frequency may possibly require prophylactic interventions (see Table 8–2). Agents customarily employed for abortive therapy include isometheptene mucate (a sympathomimetic amine used to constrict dilated cranial and cerebral arterioles), ergotamines, triptans, NSAIDs, and, in refractory cases, intravenous lidocaine. Isometheptene is fairly well tolerated, producing fewer gastrointestinal side effects that often accompany other interventions. NSAIDs might be poorly tolerated, because they can aggravate the nausea and vomiting that often accompany migraine. Sumatriptan has high efficacy and quick onset when administered subcutaneously but works more slowly when administered by intranasal or oral routes. However, the effectiveness of subcutaneous sumatriptan is brief, often necessitating a repeated dose. Generally, sumatriptan, rizatriptan, and zolmitriptan are rapidly effective but short-acting agents. If a longer duration of analgesia is required, a longer-acting triptan (e.g., eletriptan, frovatriptan, naratriptan), can be employed (Goadsby 1998; Goadsby et al. 2002).

Prophylactic headache treatment strategies are listed in Table 8–2. The pharmacologic agents listed are intended to reduce the morbidity and disability associated with recurrent migraine headache. Agents with moderate to high efficacy with minimal side effects include amitriptyline, divalproex sodium, gabapentin, propranolol, and timolol (Silberstein 2000).

Among psychotherapeutic interventions, relaxation training, biofeedback, and CBT are all somewhat effective in the prophylaxis of migraine headache (Campbell et al. 2002). However, no one modality has been demonstrated to be any more efficacious in migraine headache than any other. Certainly, integrated or combination modalities might prove to be effective for some patients (Lake 2001).

Cluster Headache

Cluster headache is significantly less common than either tension headache or migraine headache. Gender is a factor in cluster headache, with a marked prevalence among males. Cluster headache begins in one's 30s or 40s. The pain occurs in a series of attacks spanning weeks to months, with pain-free intervals of months to years. During the active period, headache can occur daily or every other day. Typically, the pain is unilateral, located in the ocular, frontal, and/or temporal areas (Welch 2001). The headache can last anywhere from 30 minutes to 2 hours, and the pain can be severe and excruciating, often arising 2–3 hours after retiring or resulting in early morning awakening. Associated features include conjunctival injection, lacrimation, stuffiness of the nose on the affected side, rhinorrhea, and ipsilateral ptosis and miosis.

Alcohol use and increased altitude are possible precipitants of cluster headache. Treatment (see Table 8–2) includes oxygen as the primary abortive agent, applied at 10 L/minute via nasal cannula. Prophylactic interventions can include ergotamines, calcium channel blockers, divalproex, methysergide, and lithium carbonate. Although lithium (600–900 mg daily) has been employed in the prophylaxis of chronic cluster headache, a double-blind, placebo-controlled trial found that lithium was not effective for prophylaxis of episodic cluster headache (Steiner et al. 1997). In such cases, calcium channel blockers or corticosteroids may be better alternatives. Note that the combination of lithium and NSAIDs would be deleterious, raising the risk of severe lithium toxicity. Clearly, avoidance of alcohol can constitute a prophylactic intervention.

Back Pain

Back pain has become one of the most common, and simultaneously one of the most elusive, chronic pain disorders. Estimates suggest that United States health care costs expended for low back pain approximate $50 billion annu-

Table 8–5. Common causes of back pain

Intervertebral disc rupture or herniation
Meningeal irritation
    Infection
    Tumor
    Bleeding
Arachnoiditis
Trauma
Prior back surgery
Facet injury
Lumbar ligament injury
Neoplasm
Spinal cord involvement (extremely dangerous)
Cauda equina syndrome (extremely dangerous)

ally. Without a doubt, back pain results in significant morbidity and constitutes the leading cause of long-term disability in the United States (Atlas and Deyo 2001).

Clinicians treating patients with back pain often are confronted with a perplexing differential diagnosis. Common causes of back pain include those listed in Table 8–5. Back pain may emanate from injury in a number of body areas (e.g., the vertebrae, facet joints, nerve roots, muscle, connective tissue). In 60% of back pain patients, there is often no direct relationship between physical findings discovered on physical examination or diagnostic testing and the patient's perceived level of pain, disability, and psychological distress (Reesor and Craig 1988). Patients whose back pain appears disproportionate to the level of pathology noted on examination have a marked propensity toward depression and maladaptive cognitive patterns compared with those with clear pathology for their pain. Such patients are particularly prone to catastrophizing as a maladaptive cognitive approach.

Patients with chronic back pain often feel frustrated by their lack of relief and may feel helpless and sometimes hopeless. Negative attitudes and beliefs that these patients have that might contribute to affective associations with the pain include a sense of loss over aspects of one's life resulting from the pain. The medical system becomes a fundamental aspect of one's life, which can be perplexing and troubling to patients, who often become frustrated with ineffective treatment strategies and extensive diagnostic testing. At times, physicians may struggle with the lack of clear identifiable causes of the pain or may become frustrated with the inability to arrive at a reasonable treatment strategy. This struggle possibly may be communicated to the patient, who might perceive the physician's approach as an endorsement of not taking the patient seriously (Walker et al. 1999).

Patients with back pain have demonstrated marked back muscle tension on EMG when discussing situations that were personally distressing, compared with other patients with chronic pain or healthy control subjects. Additionally, patients with back pain have demonstrated a protracted latency to recover or resume normal back muscle tone on EMG after cessation of the discussion (Flor et al. 1985). Distress caused or exacerbated by such discussions contributes to physiologic changes that potentially aggravate back pain.

Exercise is a fundamental aspect of treatment of patients with back pain. Patients who are encouraged by their physicians to remain active and resume their usual activity levels will have reduced disability and will return to work sooner (Waddell et al. 1997). The longer patients are out of work, the harder it is for them to return (McGill 1968). Surgical intervention might be required for structural and mechanical causes (e.g., disk herniation, spinal nerve encroachment). Nerve blocks, epidural anesthetics, or spinal anesthetics might also provide relief (see Chapter 7, "Special Techniques in Pain Management," in this volume), particularly if back pain is accompanied by radicular pain.

Medications to consider for treatment of back pain are summarized in Table 8–6. Antidepressants do not appear to have any analgesic effect greater than placebo in patients with chronic back pain (Turner and Denny 1993). However, they could be useful for patients with comorbid depression or anxiety disorders that complicate the patients' coping, adaptation, and rehabilitation process (Deyo and Weinstein 2001). Brief courses of CBT have been efficacious in reducing perceived disability and facilitating return to work in patients with chronic low back pain (Turner 1996).

Nonarticular Pain Disorders

Myofascial Pain

Myofascial pain refers to a syndrome in which the patient complains of pain in nonarticular regions of the body that originates from muscle and is precipitated

Table 8–6. Treatment options for back pain

Exercise
    Flexibility exercises
    Range-of-motion exercises
    Aerobic exercises
    Muscle strengthening exercises (e.g., of abdominal muscles)
Return to activity
Medications
    Nonsteroidal anti-inflammatory drugs, acetaminophen
    Tramadol, opioid analgesics
    Antidepressants (primarily for mood disturbances)
Other interventions
    Surgery
    Spinal cord stimulation

by muscle trigger points. The nature of the pain can simulate other disorders (e.g., trigger points in trapezius and cervical muscles can produce headache pain, and those in the paravertebral muscles can produce low back pain). Identification of trigger points is essential in diagnosing myofascial pain.

Trigger points are taut bands, palpable in muscles, that are approximately 1 cm or more across and that can roll beneath or between the fingers. Taut bands of this kind can be present both in symptomatic pain–generating muscles and in nonpainful muscles. The bands are tender, producing severe radiating pain on palpation. When stimulated, the taut bands contract briskly, producing a twitch. There may be commensurate restriction in range of motion of the limb containing the affected muscles. Pathologic investigations have not consistently demonstrated specific pathologic changes associated with trigger points.

Treatment of trigger points is possible with physiotherapy, specifically stretching and passive manipulation. Heat therapy or cryotherapy (i.e., application of cold) or application of transcutaneous electrical nerve stimulation (TENS) may also be a useful adjunct to treatment.

Fibromyalgia

Fibromyalgia, by contrast, requires the presence of multiple tender points for diagnosis. These points are located on both sides of the body, above and below the waist. Failure to meet the requisite number and distribution of tender points

Table 8–7.   Diagnostic criteria for fibromyalgia

The pain is widespread and of 3 months' duration.

Pain consists of axial pain, on both the right and left sides of the body, and above and below the waist. Pain must be present in at least three segments of the body.

There must be at least 11 tender points (of the critical 18) on digital examination (approximate force of 4 kg):

    Insertion of the suboccipital muscles into the occiput

    Upper border of the midportion of the trapezius

    Muscle attachments to the medial scapular border

    Anterior aspects of the C5 and C7 intertransverse spaces

    Second rib space at the costochondral junctions (approximately 3 cm from the sternal border)

    Muscle insertions 2 cm distal to the lateral epicondyle

    Upper outer quadrant of the gluteal muscle

    Muscle attachments posterior to the greater trochanter

    Medial fat pad proximal to the knee joint

Source.   Adapted from Wolfe F, Smythe HA, Yunus MB, et al.: "The American College of Rheumatology 1990 Criteria for the Classification of Fibromyalgia: Report of the Multicenter Criteria Committee." *Arthritis and Rheumatism* 33:171, 1990. Copyright 1990 John Wiley & Sons. Used with permission.

required for fibromyalgia leads to a diagnosis of myofascial pain syndrome. Controversy surrounds the diagnosis of fibromyalgia. The American College of Rheumatology (ACR) criteria for the diagnosis of fibromyalgia are listed in Table 8–7 (Wolfe et al. 1990). Some researchers and clinicians consider the diagnostic criteria to be too restrictive, requiring identification of a specific number and location of tender points to establish the diagnosis. Yet many patients experience tender points in other regions of the body that are not included in the "acceptable" locations defined by the ACR. However, some physicians have considered fibromyalgia to be no more than a rheumatologic rubric for somatoform disorders (Hadler 1997).

The prevalence of fibromyalgia varies depending on the populations under study. In general medical clinics, the rate of fibromyalgia is approximately 5%–10%, whereas in rheumatology practices, the rate is approximately 15%. Estimates of fibromyalgia in the general population are approximately 2%. The prevalence appears to increase with age and is higher among women (3%) than men (0.5%).

Table 8–8.   Features associated with fibromyalgia

Pain
Fatigue
Disordered sleep
Cognitive dysfunction
Dizziness
Psychological distress
Restless legs syndrome
Irritable bowel syndrome
Irritable bladder
Cold intolerance
Neurally mediated hypotension

Patients with fibromyalgia suffer immensely; additional features of the disorder are summarized in Table 8–8. In addition to muscle pain, some patients may experience joint pain and stiffness. Fatigue is prominent as a result of the deconditioning that results from chronic pain and the patient's attempts to reduce pain by rest. Other factors causing or contributing to fatigue include poor sleep, depression, and accompanying endocrine abnormalities (i.e., abnormalities in the hypothalamic-pituitary axis).

Sleep disturbances are characterized by disordered, poorly restorative sleep. Patients with fibromyalgia may be characteristically light sleepers, with a propensity to frequent arousals precipitated by noise, disruptions in the environment, or psychological distress. Some patients with fibromyalgia have alpha rhythm intrusions into Stage III and Stage IV sleep (Cohen et al. 2000). During these stages, there are normally slow-wave patterns (on electroencephalogram), and it is a time when restorative functions within the body are undertaken. Alpha rhythms signal a heightened arousal and suggest easy arousability and a diminution of normal restorative functions. Alpha rhythm intrusions are not exclusive to fibromyalgia but may occur in a number of other chronic pain disorders.

Sleep disturbances can also arise from restless legs syndrome (i.e., unusual sensations such as tingling, itching, or cramping that occur in the lower extremities with reclining but that are alleviated with leg movement, stretching, or walking). Although movement provides relief, it interferes with sleep. Restless legs disturbances may occur in as many as 30% of fibromyalgia patients.

Irritable bowel symptoms (constipation, diarrhea, or alternating consti-pation and diarrhea) along with abdominal pain and distention can occur in patients with fibromyalgia. Similarly, irritable bladder (dysuria, urgency, fre-quency in the absence of urinary tract infection or cystitis) may occur.

Paradoxical hypotensive reactions may arise resulting from catecholamine surges. Venous pooling reduces ventricular filling, resulting in lowered blood pressure. The heart rate is normally increased to compensate for the reduced pressure. During catecholamine surges, ventricular contractions increase so much that the ventricles have insufficient time to fill. Vagal reflexes are initi-ated, precipitated by ventricular mechanoreceptors, leading to syncope or near-syncope experiences.

Patients with fibromyalgia commonly experience psychological distress in the form of depression and anxiety. Depression is common in patients with fibromyalgia, but the rate of fibromyalgia is not necessarily higher among de-pressed patients. Other common disorders accompanying fibromyalgia include somatization disorders and pain disorders. High rates of childhood sexual abuse are seen in patients with fibromyalgia. Such experiences might contribute to dis-turbances in coping strategies commonly encountered in these patients.

Many studies have assessed the efficacy of various treatment approaches for patients with fibromyalgia. Many of these studies, however, are limited by short durations of follow-up of treatment efficacy, inadequate blinding, and small sample sizes. A summary of treatment measures available for patients with fibromyalgia, based on the more empirically rigorous investigations available to date, is listed in Table 8–9 (Goldenberg et al. 2004). Exercise is probably the most effective treatment. A variety of exercises can be undertaken to enhance muscle tone and reduce deconditioning, and aerobic activity can improve sleep and reduce cold intolerance. However, high-impact activities (e.g., jogging) may exacerbate pain, and thus low-impact exercises (e.g., elliptical exercise machines) might be better tolerated. Treatment of pain may be attempted with the use of antidepressants, which may also reduce comorbid depression. Low doses of antidepressant are generally required for pain, whereas the usual antidepressant doses might be required for comorbid mood or anxiety disorders. Some clinicians advocate the use of tramadol, and opiate analgesics might be re-quired, at least temporarily. Treatment options for associated features of fibro-myalgia (e.g., restless legs syndrome) are listed in Table 8–10.

Table 8–9.   Summary of treatment approaches for fibromyalgia based on strength of evidence in the available literature

Strength of evidence	Pharmacologic	Nonpharmacologic
Strong	Amitriptyline	Cardiovascular exercise
	Cyclobenzaprine	CBT
		Group educational sessions
Moderate	Tramadol±acetaminophen	Strength training
	Fluoxetine	Acupuncture
	Duloxetine	Biofeedback
	Venlafaxine	Hypnosis
	Milnacipran	
	Pregabalin	
Weak	Growth hormone	Massage
	5-Hydroxytryptamine	Ultrasound
	S-Adenosylmethionine	Chiropractic therapy
No evidence	Opioids	Tender point injections
	NSAIDs	
	Benzodiazepines	
	Thyroid hormone	
	Calcitonin	
	Dehydroepiandrosterone	
	Magnesium	

Note.   Strength of evidence for treatment efficacy: strong=positive results from a meta-analysis or from more than one randomized controlled trial (RCT); moderate=positive results from one RCT, largely positive results from multiple RCTs, or consistently positive results from multiple non-RCTs; weak=positive results from descriptive and case studies, inconsistent results from RCTs, or both. CBT=cognitive-behavioral therapy; NSAID=nonsteroidal anti-inflammatory drug.
Source.   Adapted with permission from Goldenberg DL, Burckhardt C, Crofford L: "Management of Fibromyalgia Syndrome." *Journal of the American Medical Association* 292:2388–2395, 2004. Copyright 2004, American Medical Association.

A multidisciplinary approach to pain management is advocated for patients with fibromyalgia. Involvement of psychiatrists, rheumatologists, and physiatrists might best lead to a comprehensive treatment approach. Group therapy can be very helpful for these patients. The context of such groups may reduce the sense of isolation that can occur in patients with a debilitating disorder, may foster group problem solving, and allows for the sharing of effective treatment strategies among peers. Demands on medical resources could be reduced by patients' participation in such groups.

Table 8–10. Pharmacologic treatment strategies for comorbidities of fibromyalgia

Anxiolytics (for anxiety)

Antidepressants (for pain, comorbid depression)

Dopamine agonists (e.g., ropinirole, pramipexole, carbidopa-levodopa 10/100 at bedtime [first choice for restless legs syndrome]); clonazepam 0.5–1.0 mg at bedtime is an alternative for restless legs syndrome

Serotonin (5-HT$_4$) agonists (e.g., tegaserod [for constipation-type irritable bowel])

Serotonin (5-HT$_3$) antagonists (e.g., alosetron [for diarrhea-type irritable bowel])

Antispasmodics (e.g., Donnatal or dicyclomine [for irritable bowel syndrome] or oxybutynin [for irritable bladder])

Fludrocortisone (for neurally mediated hypotension)

Sedative-hypnotics

Osteoarthritis and Rheumatoid Arthritis

In addition to the nonarticular rheumatologic conditions discussed previously, a number of articular disorders warrant the attention of the pain specialist. Among these, osteoarthritis and rheumatoid arthritis are among the most common. In the United States, as many as 40 million persons are affected by arthritis and musculoskeletal conditions.

Osteoarthritis (degenerative joint disease) is the most common form of arthritis and is the most prevalent articular disease affecting elderly persons. The condition results from destruction of joint cartilage by chondrocytes and affects multiple joints, including the distal interphalangeal joints, the proximal interphalangeal joints, spine, hip, and knees, but rarely wrist, shoulder, or metacarpal-phalangeal joints. Weight-bearing joints are most apt to be affected. Osteoarthritis may arise from primary joint dysfunction, involving the synovial capsule, or it can arise from secondary processes (e.g., prior injury or joint trauma). Symptoms of osteoarthritis can be very distressing and may include pain, joint stiffness (especially after inactivity), swelling, deformity, and ultimate loss of function. Because of joint degeneration, osteoarthritis causes significant morbidity, accounting for substantial work disability in persons over age 50 years.

Treatment endeavors should include weight loss, exercise (especially of the knee joints), and analgesics. Weight loss becomes difficult for many patients, par-

Table 8–11. Treatment options for patients with osteoarthritis

Medication
  Celecoxib
  Nonsteroidal anti-inflammatory drugs
  Steroids
Topical agents
  Capsaicin
  Methyl salicylate creams
Intra-articular injections
  Glucocorticoids
  Hyaluronic acid
Nonpharmacologic interventions
  Physical therapy
  Weight loss
  Surgical management
    Arthroplasty
    Arthroscopic removal of loose bodies
    Correction of anatomic defects (spondylosis, spinal stenosis)
Emerging trends
  Exogenous growth factors (to stimulate chondrocyte proliferation)
  Transplantation of healthy chondrocytes, engineered to maximally produce
    growth factors

ticularly because patients tend to minimize activity levels so as to avoid pain. Thus, they run the risk of becoming deconditioned and less capable of sustaining aerobic activity and physical fitness. Pain relief can be brought forth by any of the NSAIDs. Celecoxib might be better tolerated because of its reduced propensity to interfere with gastric and renal functioning (see also Chapter 5, "Pharmacology of Pain," of this book for adverse effects associated with NSAIDs and cyclooxygenase-2 inhibitors). These and other medications to employ in the treatment of osteoarthritis are summarized in Table 8–11.

Rheumatoid arthritis, on the other hand, is an inflammatory process affecting the synovium of articular joints and producing a number of systemic manifestations. Rheumatoid arthritis affects approximately 1%–2% of the population, with about two to three times as many women affected as men. The joints affected by rheumatoid arthritis include the hands, wrists, elbows, ankles,

Table 8–12. Treatment options for patients with rheumatoid arthritis

Anti-inflammatory agents
    Nonsteroidal anti-inflammatory drugs
    Celecoxib
    Corticosteroids
Disease modifying antirheumatic drugs
    Leflunomide
    Soluble interleukin-1 receptor therapy
        Anakinra
    Tumor necrosis factor inhibitors
        Etanercept
        Infliximab
    Methotrexate
    Hydroxychloroquine
    Sulfasalazine
    Intramuscular gold
    Cytotoxic agents
        Cyclosporin A
        Azathioprine
        Cyclophosphamide

feet, and cervical spine. The joints may be swollen and tender, and over time there occur significant deformities of the hands, including ulnar deviation and the swan-neck and boutonniere deformities of the fingers. Patients with rheumatoid arthritis experience a number of systemic problems arising from the inflammatory processes of the disease, including subcutaneous nodules, anemia, vasculitic processes, entrapment neuropathy, interstitial nephritis, and effusions (pericardial and pleural). Treatment endeavors directed at patients with rheumatoid arthritis are listed in Table 8–12.

Because there is so much loss, disability, and discomfort accompanying arthritic conditions, it is not surprising that significant mood disturbances can accompany the disorder. Depression appears to be the most prevalent psychological disturbance accompanying osteoarthritis and rheumatoid arthritis. Pain severity among patients with arthritis was found to be correlated with the presence of depression—higher among those who were depressed, compared with nondepressed patients or those with only a remote history of depression (Frank et al. 1988). The relationship between pain severity and mood disturbances is not exclusive to depression, however. Ratings of pain severity have also been associated with other unpleasant emotional states, such as anger and anxiety (Huyser and Parker 1999). In addition, functional impairments and perceived disability associated with arthritic conditions are likewise related to these emotional states. Depression and anxiety may interfere with treatment adherence (e.g., lack of participation in an exercise program and weight loss). Consequently, psychopharmacologic agents, although not directly analgesic in arthritic conditions, may indirectly reduce emotional distress and perceived functional impairments and thereby reduce perceived pain severity and facilitate treatment.

Psychological variables may mediate levels of pain and disability as well. Cognitive approaches—including a propensity to catastrophize, overgeneralize, or selectively abstract—appear to be related to perceived levels of distress and disability associated with arthritic conditions (Smith et al. 1988). Patients with passive coping strategies (e.g., wishful thinking, self-blame) have been found to have poorer functional abilities than those with more active, problem-solving approaches (Young 1992). Thus, psychotherapies (e.g., CBT) might be particularly advantageous in improving functional adaptations in patients with arthritic conditions by addressing cognitive distortions and fostering improved coping strategies.

Neuropathic Pain

Neuropathic pain is often confusing, in part because the causes of neuropathic pain are often unclear. In addition, treatment of neuropathic pain can be difficult, and the pain can progress to the point of causing complete disability. Consequently, patients and physicians alike can be frustrated with neuropathic pain, being overwhelmed by its effects and disgruntled with its relatively refractory quality.

Neuropathic pain is associated with features of unusual sensations in an area of the body that intensify over the course of the day and over time. Typically, patients describe the pain as constant burning or electric in quality in a body area that was previously injured but that demonstrates no ongoing damage (Rowbotham 1995). The pain often emanates from areas of the body that on physical examination demonstrate sensory loss. The condition is characterized by allodynia (i.e., pain produced by normally nonnoxious stimulation) and hyperpathia (i.e., exaggerated pain response to a noxious stimulus). At times, physical signs commensurate with sympathetic nervous system involvement are present.

Neuropathic pain can arise from a number of sources (see Table 8–13). Aδ and C fibers are neurons responsible for mediation of pain (see Chapter 2, "Sensory Pathways of Pain and Acute Versus Chronic Pain," of this book). Processes that may aggravate the pain-relaying Aδ and C fibers include nerve impingement (e.g., carpal tunnel syndrome, tumor impingement on brachial or lumbar plexus, disk herniation compressing adjacent nerve roots). Trigeminal neuralgia is attributed to localized compression of the trigeminal nerve by neighboring vascular structures. For these conditions, nerve conduction studies might reveal delays in the conduction velocities between the affected (painful) side and the unaffected side. The EMG might also reveal concomitant weakness when the motor components of the nerve are adversely affected. Computed tomography or magnetic resonance imaging may detect the affected nerves. Treatment is directed at relieving the underlying compression or nerve irritation (e.g., decompression of the median nerve, use of anticancer drugs, radiation therapy, splinting the affected limb, use of corticosteroids). Nerves that are damaged by illness or trauma can lead to firing of neurons at ectopic sites in a way that relays pain. For example, large-diameter fibers (A fibers) are damaged in disease states such as diabetes mellitus; when this happens, C fibers fire unabatedly, relaying chronic pain in the distribution of the affected nerve.

Peripheral nociceptors relay information from the skin, joints, muscles, bone, organs, and so forth. The fibers synapse on second-order neurons within the spinal cord. These, in turn, relay information to third-order neurons within the thalamus. Damage to peripheral fibers can actually lead to spontaneous firing in second- or third-order neurons in the pain-mediating process. This firing may be perceived as painful. Central nervous system lesions (e.g., stroke, arteriovascular malformations) may also produce pain in the pain transmission pathway.

Treatment strategies employed for neuropathic states are summarized in Table 8–14 (see also Chapter 5 of this book). The mainstays of treatment include TCAs, anticonvulsants, antiarrhythmics, and topical agents (Argoff et

Table 8–13. Sources of neuropathic pain

Anatomic conditions causing neuropathy
  Entrapment neuropathy (carpal tunnel syndrome, ulnar entrapment, others)
  Trigeminal neuralgia
Medical conditions causing neuropathy
  Diabetic neuropathy
  HIV-related neuropathy
  Malignancy
  Postherpetic neuralgia
  Rheumatologic conditions producing neuropathy (rheumatoid arthritis, Sjögren's syndrome, systemic lupus erythematosus)
Toxin-induced neuropathy
  Alcohol
  Arsenic
  Cisplatin
  Dideoxynucleoside
  Paclitaxel
  Vincristine
Guillain-Barré syndrome
Fabry's disease
Vasculitic neuropathy
Amyloid neuropathy
Idiopathic distal small-fiber neuropathy

al. 2006; Galer 1995; Leo 2006). Treatment should be initiated early in the course of illness for optimal results (e.g., when amitriptyline is initiated within 3 months of developing the rash of herpes zoster infection, patients are less likely to develop the complications of postherpetic neuralgia) (Bowsher 1997). Restriction of and delays in the efficacy of TCAs in producing analgesia would be expected if they are administered after significant peripheral and central pathophysiologic mechanisms have set in. There are emerging data suggesting that anticonvulsants (e.g., pregabalin, gabapentin) may likewise have a preemptive analgesic role (Dahl et al. 2004). Other treatment interventions that may mitigate the pain experience include TENS, biofeedback, relaxation training, and hypnosis.

Table 8–14. Treatment strategies for patients with neuropathic pain

Anticonvulsants	Gabapentin 900–3,600 mg/day
	Pregabalin 300–600 mg/day
	Carbamazepine 600–1,200 mg/day
	Divalproex sodium 750–2,500 mg/day
	Clonazepam 0.5–3 mg/day
Opiates	Methadone 5–100 mg/day
	Oxycodone controlled-release 10–60 mg q 12 hours
	Tramadol 50–400 mg/day
Antidepressants	Duloxetine 60–120 mg/day
	Amitriptyline 25–200 mg/day
	Nortriptyline 25–150 mg/day
	Desipramine 25–200 mg/day
Other medications	Mexiletine 450–900 mg/day
	Dexamethasone 6–100 mg/day
	Topical capsaicin
	Topical lidocaine (5% patch)
Other interventions	Transcutaneous electrical nerve stimulation
	Sympathetic nerve blocks
	Epidural and intrathecal nerve blocks
	Nerve ablation
	Cordotomy, rhizotomy
	Spinal stimulation
	Hypnosis, biofeedback, relaxation training

Sympathetically Mediated Pain: Complex Regional Pain Syndromes

Complex regional pain syndromes (CRPSs) comprise two types of disorders: CRPS I (previously referred to as reflex sympathetic dystrophy) and CRPS II (previously referred to as causalgia). CRPS I results from some inciting event, often a traumatic, infectious, or vascular event within soft tissue, whereas CRPS II arises from direct nerve injury (Bonica 1973). In either case, the inciting event induces a series of responses that are mediated by the sympathetic nervous system. If these conditions are untreated or unabated, the sympathetic nervous system responses produce marked trophic changes in a limb.

The most prominent feature of CRPS is pain, often throbbing (for CRPS I) or burning (for CRPS II). The pain is usually constant, but paroxysms of pain can occur, ranging from mild to severe. Initially, the pain is often located at the site of injury, but it can extend through the entire affected limb. Over time, there can be extension of pain to other limbs unaffected by the initial trauma or injury. The affected limb is often exquisitely sensitive to ambient temperature, touch, or stimulation associated with movement. Thus, the patient will tend to guard the painful limb and withdraw from physical examination that could raise the risk of pain from touch or direct manipulation. In addition, there are a number of changes in temperature, skin, muscle tone, vascular system, and bone that occur as the course of the disorder progresses. Classic features of CRPS include changes in blood flow within, along with resultant temperature changes in, the affected limb as compared with other limbs; edema; and trophic skin changes, along with changes in the musculature and changes in bone scan activity and density. The rate of progression of the changes associated with CRPS varies from person to person.

Several investigations may be employed to assess the features and staging of CRPS. For example, skin temperature depends on the extent of cutaneous blood flow, which is under the direct influence of sympathetic activity. In early stages of CRPS, thermography may reveal increased temperature in the affected limb compared with the contralateral limb or other limbs of the body. In later stages, skin blood flow and temperature are reduced. Bone scanning by scintigraphy may reveal increased activity throughout the bones of the affected limb. Bone density measurements may reveal progressive changes in the bone of the affected limb over time.

Treatment approaches for CRPS include pharmacologic treatment (see Table 8–15). A number of invasive techniques may be employed as well, given the relatively refractory nature of such syndromes to pharmacologic approaches. Nerve blocks may be employed to disrupt ongoing sympathetic nervous system activity in the affected limb. Surgical interventions to disrupt sympathetic nervous system activity may be employed (sympathectomy) for patients who are unable to sustain extended relief from repeated nerve blocks.

Affective disorders are common among patients with CRPS—for example, more than 60% of patients meet criteria for major depression (Galer et al.

Table 8–15.   Treatment of patients with complex regional pain syndrome

Medications
    Anticonvulsants (carbamazepine, phenytoin, gabapentin, pregabalin)
    Antidepressants (tricyclic antidepressants)
    Baclofen (oral/intrathecal)
    Calcium channel blockers
    Clonidine (oral/intrathecal)
    Corticosteroids (chronic use is not recommended)
    Lidocaine patch
    Opioids
    Phenoxybenzamine
    Prazosin
    Propranolol
Local nerve block
Regional sympathetic block (cervical, lumbar)
Sympathectomy
Spinal cord stimulation (implantable device)
Physical therapy

2001). Substance abuse disorders also are common among this population. There is controversy about whether premorbid psychological disturbances predispose one to CRPS. In any event, psychiatric treatment for these conditions is warranted. Biofeedback and relaxation training can reduce distress and foster adaptive strategies with which to deal with pain (Barowsky et al. 1987).

Phantom Limb Pain

After amputation, it is common for patients to experience sensations of the removed limb, just as though it were present (phantom sensations). In some cases, these sensations progress to distressing painful sensations (phantom pain) perceived to be emanating from the amputated limb.

Although phantom limb sensations are almost universal following amputation, approximately 85%–97% of amputees experience some form of pain. Sensations are almost immediate, whereas pain might not emerge for some time after amputation, typically from 1 month to 1 year. Pain is often characterized as burning, cramping, or aching. Other features (e.g., crushing, squeezing, twisting, pins and needles, grinding) are also described (Jensen et al. 1985). Pain may be exacerbated by physical stimulation and emotional factors (e.g., depression). The characteristics of phantom limb pain can vary widely in terms of the quality of sensory experiences and impact on quality of life. Thus, in the mildest forms of phantom limb pain, patients may experience mild, intermittent paresthesias that do not interfere with normal activity or sleep; in extreme forms, paresthesias may be constant and very uncomfortable, interfering with activity and sleep.

The course of phantom limb pain is variable, with up to 56% of patients reporting resolution or improvement in symptoms over time. Pain emerging over time warrants investigation of possible causes producing pain (e.g., infection at the site of amputation, scar tissue, neuroma formation). The cause of phantom pain is unclear. Peripheral processes (i.e., spontaneous discharges emanating from severed nerves containing Aδ and C fibers) brought on by scar tissue in the amputated limb are thought to be a possible basis of this pain. Spontaneous discharges such as these may be inhibited by infusions of lidocaine but could be exacerbated by irritation of the stump (e.g., tapping) or cold exposure. Alternatively, central processes (i.e., reverberating neural circuits within the central nervous system) have also been implicated as the basis for phantom limb pain.

Specific psychological correlates of persons experiencing phantom limb pain are lacking. However, some data tend to suggest that among those experiencing this form of pain, there is a tendency to be rigid, inflexible, and self-reliant; to suppress emotions (thus depriving one of the propensity to grieve the lost limb); and to cope by using denial as a primary defense. It is theorized that phantom limb pain possibly may arise from psychopathologic interpretations of phantom limb sensations (Parkes 1973).

Treatment for patients with phantom limb pain may include antidepressants and anticonvulsants (Hord 1996). However, controlled studies on the efficacy of such agents are generally lacking; efficacy has been based mostly on anecdotal reports. Another group of agents, β-blockers, may also reduce phantom limb pain and may be considered as alternatives to, or used in conjunction with, antidepressants and anticonvulsants. Opiates tend not to be effective for long-term use in phantom limb pain.

Surgical interventions have been employed in the past for phantom limb pain but, because of their limited utility, have largely been abandoned (e.g., thalamotomy, sympathectomy, cordotomy). Neurolytic and sympathetic blocks might be useful in selected patients. Epidural anesthesia administered for 3 days prior to the amputation may reduce the severity of postoperative phantom limb pain (Bach et al. 1988). Psychological therapies (e.g., relaxation training) possibly may help to reduce the distress associated with the pain and help to reduce the pain sensations. Psychotherapy might be required to help the patient mourn the loss of the limb, address concerns over physical appearance or disfigurement, and facilitate adaptation to the use of prostheses and making the changes necessary to modify his or her usual activities.

Cancer and HIV

Pain complicates the clinical picture of approximately 50% of patients with metastatic cancer (Ahles et al. 1983). The nature of the pain—its location, intensity, radiation, quality, and other characteristics—may vary depending on the type of cancer, its progression, and the treatment measures undertaken to treat it.

Among patients with HIV/AIDS, prevalence rates for pain vary from 30% to 97%. The variability in prevalence rates of pain associated with HIV is in part attributable to the progression of the disease and the clinical settings in which patient evaluations were conducted (Breitbart and Patt 1994). Common pain-related disorders associated with HIV/AIDS (Lebovits et al. 1989) are summarized in Table 8–16.

Pain ratings for patients with cancer are higher among those with comorbid psychiatric conditions than in those without such conditions (Massie and Holland 1987). Common psychiatric comorbidity includes adjustment disorders, depression, anxiety, and delirium.

Effective pain treatment is obviously contingent on the nature and source of pain (Benedetti et al. 2000). Thus, opioids might be required for severe bone pain due to metastases, fractures, or both; antidepressants, anticonvulsants, or both may be employed in neuropathic types of pains. Pharmacologic approaches to pain management (see Table 8–17) need to be customized to the patient's needs, factoring pain severity, impact on functioning, and tolerability of side effects. Anti-inflammatory agents are required for mild pain, but opioids might be required for moderate to severe pain states. Dosing sched-

Table 8–16.   Common pain-related disorders associated with HIV/AIDS

Nociceptive

Cutaneous

   Kaposi sarcoma

   Oral cavity pain

  Candidiasis

  Aphthous ulcers

  Herpes simplex virus and cytomegalovirus infection

Visceral

   Ulcerative esophagitis

   Gastritis

   Pancreatitis and biliary tract disorders

   Tumor

   Infection

Deep somatic

   Arthralgias

   Back pain

   Myopathies

Headache

   Meningitis

   Encephalitis

   Iatrogenic causes (e.g., zidovudine)

Neuropathic

Mononeuropathy

Guillain-Barré syndrome

Mononeuropathy multiplex

Polyneuropathy

Herpes simplex (postherpetic neuralgia)

Antiretroviral toxicity–associated neuropathy

ules should be simple to maximize adherence and should be administered in the least invasive manner. Persistent pain requires around-the-clock dosing of analgesics. Certainly psychiatric interventions, including pharmacotherapy and psychotherapy, are prudent in conditions in which there is psychiatric comorbidity. Adjunctive techniques (e.g., hypnosis, relaxation training, bio-

Table 8–17.   Management of cancer pain and pain associated with HIV and AIDS, based on pain ratings

Mild (1–3)	Consider nonsteroidal anti-inflammatory drug, acetaminophen
	If ineffective, augment with opiate
	If ineffective, administer short-acting opiate
Moderate (4–6)	Consider short-acting opiate
	Consider augmentation of opiates with psychotropics
	Address side effects of opiates (gastrointestinal side effects, sedation, delirium)
Severe (7–10)	Consider rapid dose increases of short-acting opiate
	5–10 mg morphine (or equivalent)
	Reassess after 1 hour
	Double the dose if pain is unchanged; reassess after 1 hour
	Repeat dose if pain level is halved; reassess after 1 hour
	If improved (pain is less than 50% of original level), reassess after 1 hour
	Give the effective dose administered after 4 hours, then give this dose every 4 hours around the clock
	Consider augmentation of opiates with psychotropics
	Address side effects of opiates (gastrointestinal side effects, sedation, delirium)

Note.   Pain ratings are based on a numeric rating scale of 1–10.

feedback, deep breathing exercises) might facilitate mitigation of pain and accompanying psychological distress. However, the presence of an underlying delirium would certainly limit the ability of the patient to obtain any benefit from psychotherapeutic interventions. In such cases, resolution of the underlying medical condition, the addition of antipsychotics, or both, might be required to reduce the interference of any psychological interventions by a delirium.

The attributions assigned to the pain by the cancer patient may be the basis for a great deal of psychological distress. It is not uncommon for the patient to ascribe ominous interpretations to the presence of the pain, which in turn could exacerbate the pain experience. However, such attributions that pain could signal disease progression might not be entirely unrealistic (Ahles et al. 1983). Other sources of distress may include immediate concrete needs (e.g., financial needs, housing, transportation), family or interpersonal concerns, changes in one's autonomy and independence, need for assistance with activities of daily living, and spiritual concerns (e.g., afterlife issues, making amends, mending interpersonal conflicts). Such issues, once identified, might require the joint efforts of the psychiatrist, psychologist, social worker, and pastoral counselor for effective management (Holland 1999).

Key Points

- For many chronic, nonmalignant pain conditions, the goals of treatment include symptomatic pain control, improvement in function, and reduction of disability, along with management of comorbidities (e.g., sleep disturbances, fatigue, mood disturbances).
- Primary headache disorders are highly prevalent conditions. Successful management requires accurate diagnosis, recognition of appropriate treatment modalities available, and management of common comorbidities.
- Back pain is a common cause of pain and disability. For many patients with nonemergent, nonspecific back pain, treatment directed at reassurance, exercise, use of weak analgesics, and psychotherapeutic interventions may be all that is necessary.
- Fibromyalgia is characterized by widespread nonarticular pain. It is often associated with fatigue, sleep disturbances, restless legs syndrome, irritable bowel symptoms, and hypotension. A multidisciplinary approach employing prudent pharmacologic interventions, graded exercise programs, patient education, and cognitive-behavioral therapy can address symptoms and improve functioning.
- Treatment of articular disorders (e.g., osteoarthritis, rheumatoid arthritis) necessitates pharmacologic interventions, physical/occupational therapies, ambulatory/assistive devices, and, in some cases, surgical interventions. Psychological comorbidities can contribute to distress by magnifying pain, enhancing perceived disability, and undermining treatment and rehabilitative interventions and may warrant intervention.
- Although neuropathic pain can arise from an array of etiologies, several effective treatment modalities are available that mitigate peripheral and central

nervous system processes that enhance pain. The mainstays of treatment include tricyclic antidepressants, anticonvulsants, antiarrhythmics, and topical agents.

- Pain related to cancer and HIV is multifactorial—that is, due to the primary illness and comorbid illnesses and conditions, and due to the treatment itself—warranting aggressive treatment. Such pain can be magnified by psychological and spiritual distress.

References

Ahles TA, Blanchard EB, Ruckdeschel JC: The multidimensional nature of cancer-related pain. Pain 17:277–288, 1983

Ansari A: The efficacy of newer antidepressants in the treatment of chronic pain: a review of current literature. Harv Rev Psychiatry 7:257–277, 2000

Argoff CE, Backonja MM, Belgrade MJ, et al: Consensus guidelines: treatment planning and options. Mayo Clin Proc 81 (suppl 4):12–25, 2006

Atlas SJ, Deyo RA: Evaluating and managing acute low back pain in the primary care setting. J Gen Intern Med 16:120–131, 2001

Bach S, Noreng MF, Tjellden NU: Phantom limb pain in amputees during the first 12 months following limb amputation, after preoperative lumbar epidural blockade. Pain 33:297–301, 1988

Barowsky EI, Zweig JB, Moskowitz J: Thermal biofeedback in the treatment of symptoms associated with reflex sympathetic dystrophy. J Child Neurol 2:229–232, 1987

Bendtsen L, Jensen R: Mirtazapine is effective in the prophylactic treatment of chronic tension-type headache. Neurology 62:1706–1711, 2004

Benedetti C, Brock C, Cleeland C, et al: NCCN practice guidelines for cancer pain. Oncology 14:135–150, 2000

Bogaards MC, ter Kuile MM: Treatment of recurrent tension headache: a meta-analytic review. Clin J Pain 10:174–190, 1994

Bonica JJ: Causalgia and other reflex sympathetic dystrophies. Postgrad Med 53:143–148, 1973

Bowsher D: The effects of pre-emptive treatment of postherpetic neuralgia with amitriptyline: a randomized, double-blind, placebo-controlled trial. J Pain Symptom Manage 13:327–331, 1997

Breitbart W, Patt RB: Pain management in the patient with AIDS. Hem/Onc Annals: The Journal of Continuing Education in Hematology and Oncology 2:391–399, 1994

Breslau N, Lipton RB, Stewart WF, et al: Comorbidity of migraine and depression: investigating potential etiology and prognosis. Neurology 60:1308–1312, 2003

Campbell JK, Penzien DB, Wall EM: Evidence-based guidelines for migraine headache: behavioral and physical treatments. The U.S. Headache Consortium. Available at: http://www.aan.com/professionals/practice/pdfs/gL0089.pdf. Accessed June 2002.

Cohen MJM, Menefee LA, Doghramji K, et al: Sleep in chronic pain: problems and treatments. Int Rev Psychiatry 12:115–127, 2000

Collins JG: Prevalence of selected chronic conditions, United States, 1979–1981. Data from the National Health Survey. Vital Health Stat 10:1–66, 1986

Dahl JB, Mathiesen O, Moiniche S: "Protective premedication": an option with gabapentin and related drugs? A review of gabapentin and pregabalin in the treatment of post-operative pain. Acta Anaesthesiol Scand 48:1130–1136, 2004

Deyo RA, Weinstein JN: Low back pain. N Engl J Med 344:363–370, 2001

Diamond S: Efficacy and safety profile of venlafaxine in chronic headache. Headache Quarterly, Current Treatment and Research 6:212–214, 1995

Epstein MT, Hockaday JM, Hockaday TDR: Migraine and reproductive hormones throughout the menstrual cycle. Lancet 1:543–548, 1975

Fasmer OB: The prevalence of migraine in patients with bipolar and unipolar affective disorders. Cephalalgia 21:894–899, 2001

Flor H, Turk DC, Birbaumer N: Assessment of stress-related psychophysiological reactions in chronic back pain patients. J Consult Clin Psychol 53:354–364, 1985

Frank RG, Beck NC, Parker JC, et al: Depression in rheumatoid arthritis. J Rheumatol 15:920–925, 1988

Galer BS: Neuropathic pain of peripheral origin: advances in pharmacologic treatment. Neurology 45 (suppl 9):17–25, 1995

Galer BS, Schwartz L, Allen RJ: Complex regional pain syndromes, type I: reflex sympathetic dystrophy, and type II: causalgia, in Bonica's Management of Pain, 3rd Edition. Edited by Loeser JD, Butler SH, Chapman CR, et al. Philadelphia, PA, Lippincott Williams & Wilkins, 2001, pp 388–411

Goadsby PJ: Serotonin 5-HT$_{1B/1D}$ receptor agonists in migraine: comparative pharmacology and its therapeutic implications. CNS Drugs 10:271–286, 1998

Goadsby PJ, Lipton RB, Ferrari MD: Migraine: current understanding and treatment. N Engl J Med 346:257–270, 2002

Goldenberg DL, Burckhardt C, Crofford L: Management of fibromyalgia syndrome. JAMA 292:2388–2395, 2004

Hadler NM: Fibromyalgia, chronic fatigue, and other iatrogenic diagnostic algorithms. Postgrad Med 102:161–177, 1997

Holland JC: Update: NCCN practice guidelines for the management of psychosocial distress. Oncology 13:459–507, 1999

Holm JE, Holroyd KA, Hursey KG, et al: The role of stress in recurrent tension headache. Headache 26:160–167, 1986

Holroyd KA, Andrasik F, Westbrook T: Cognitive control of tension headache. Cognit Ther Res 1:121–133, 1977

Holroyd KA, O'Donnell FJ, Stensland M, et al: Management of chronic tension-type headache with tricyclic antidepressant medication, stress management therapy, and their combination. JAMA 285:2208–2215, 2001

Hord AH: Phantom pain, in Pain Management: A Comprehensive Review. Edited by Raj PP. St Louis, MO, Mosby, 1996, pp 483–491

Huyser BA, Parker JC: Negative affect and pain in arthritis. Rheum Dis Clin North Am 25:105–121, 1999

Jensen TS, Krebs B, Nielsen J, et al: Immediate and long-term phantom limb pain in amputees: incidence, clinical characteristics and relationship to pre-amputation limb pain. Pain 21:267–278, 1985

Lake AE 3rd: Behavioral and nonpharmacologic treatments of headache. Med Clin North Am 85:1055–1075, 2001

Lebovits AH, Lefkowitz M, McCarthy D, et al: The prevalence and management of pain in patients with AIDS: a review of 134 cases. Clin J Pain 5:245–248, 1989

Leo RJ: Treatment considerations in neuropathic pain. Curr Treat Options Neurol 8:389–400, 2006

Lipchik GL, Nash JM: Cognitive-behavioral issues in the treatment and management of chronic daily headache. Curr Pain Headache Rep 6:473–479, 2002

Massie MJ, Holland JC: The cancer patient with pain: psychiatric complications and their management. Med Clin North Am 71:243–258, 1987

McGill CM: Industrial back problems: a control program. J Occup Med 10:174–178, 1968

Parkes CM: Factors determining the persistence of phantom pain in the amputee. J Psychosom Res 17:97–108, 1973

Reesor KA, Craig KD: Medically incongruent chronic back pain: physical limitations, suffering, and ineffective coping. Pain 32:35–45, 1988

Rowbotham MC: Chronic pain: from theory to practical management. Neurology 45 (suppl 9):5–10, 1995

Saper JR, Lake AE, Tepper SJ: Nefazodone for chronic daily headache prophylaxis: an open-label study. Headache 41:465–474, 2001

Silberstein SD: The role of sex hormones in headache. Neurology 42 (suppl 2):37–42, 1992

Silberstein SD: Practice parameter: evidence-based guidelines for migraine headache (an evidence-based review): report of the Quality Standards Subcommittee of the American Academy of Neurology. Neurology 55:754–762, 2000

Smith TW, Peck JR, Milano RA, et al: Cognitive distortion in rheumatoid arthritis: relation to depression and disability. J Consult Clin Psychol 56:412–416, 1988

Steiner TJ, Hering R, Couturier EG, et al: Double-blind placebo-controlled trial of lithium in episodic cluster headache. Cephalalgia 17:673–675, 1997

Stewart WF, Ricci JA, Chee E, et al: Lost productive time and cost due to common pain conditions in the US workforce. JAMA 290:2443–2454, 2003

Turner JA: Educational and behavioral interventions for back pain in primary care. Spine 21:2851–2857, 1996

Turner JA, Denny MC: Do antidepressant medications relieve chronic low back pain? J Fam Pract 37:545–553, 1993

Waddell G, Feder G, Lewis M: Systematic reviews of bed rest and advice to stay active for acute low back pain. Br J Gen Pract 47:647–652, 1997

Walker J, Holloway I, Sofaer B: In the system: the lived experience of chronic back pain from the perspectives of those seeking help from pain clinics. Pain 80:621–628, 1999

Welch KMA: Headache, in Bonica's Management of Pain, 3rd Edition. Edited by Loeser JD, Butler SH, Chapman CR, et al. Philadelphia, PA, Lippincott Williams & Wilkins, 2001, pp 867–894

Wolfe F, Smythe HA, Yunus MB, et al: The American College of Rheumatology 1990 criteria for the classification of fibromyalgia: report of the Multicenter Criteria Committee. Arthritis Rheum 33:160–172, 1990

Young LD: Psychological factors in rheumatoid arthritis. J Consult Clin Psychol 60:619–627, 1992

Zwart JA, Dyb G, Hagen K, et al: Depression and anxiety disorders associated with headache frequency: the Nord-Trondelag Health Study. Eur J Neurol 10:147–152, 2003

9

Special Populations

Pain management of special populations, each with its own set of issues, can be challenging. The recognition and treatment of pain in the very young and the very old have been poor. There are fears, misconceptions, and stereotypes that have an impact on pain management among pregnant patients, culturally distinct groups, and persons with substance abuse histories. Unique issues also arise among patients with terminal conditions and their families.

Pediatric Patients

Pain management among children has been abysmally poor. For example, the level of analgesics provided to children postoperatively was markedly low compared with the level provided to adults in comparable surgical interventions (Beyer et al. 1983). Part of this poor pain management has been due to misconceptions about pediatric pain, to inadequate pain assessments and scales for use in young children, and to fears about the use of powerful analgesics (e.g., opiates) among young patients.

The neonatal nervous system is well equipped to process nociceptive input (Goldschneider et al. 2001). However, the communication of painful states is limited. Common chronic pain states in children include headache, recurrent abdominal and chest pain, and those pain states associated with chronic illnesses (e.g., diabetes, sickle cell anemia, hemophilia, juvenile rheumatoid arthritis, cancer).

Pain and Childhood Developmental Phases

Any pain management approach needs to include the psychological, cognitive, and emotional factors present at varying developmental phases appropriate to children. Among infants, pain is responded to reflexively, with expression of discomfort conveyed through crying. Facial expressions and crying patterns appear to be distinct for pain as compared with other unpleasant states (e.g., hunger) (Sifford 1997). Among toddlers, words might be expressed for pain (e.g., "ouch," "boo-boo"). However, such children are likely to view pain in terms of punishment (i.e., as an indicator of being "bad"). It is imperative that provision of pain relief be undertaken in a way that avoids fostering such misconceptions. At school age, in concrete operational ways, the child may assign emotional terms to pain. Pain is no longer viewed as punishment, and the child can assimilate cause-and-effect understanding of the pain. Differentiation among varying pain intensities becomes possible at approximately ages 5–7 years. Later, among young adults, there is a sense of invulnerability (which could account in part for the reckless behaviors that precipitate injuries warranting pain treatment). Body image, peer relations, and school attendance are central to their experiences. Thus, the presence of pain may threaten the adolescent's sense of invulnerability, separate him or her from peers, and lead to concerns about self-image and self-esteem.

Pain Assessment Scales

Pain assessments for children and adolescents need to be appropriate to developmental stage, and suitable assessment scales can be helpful. In infants and preverbal children, the emphasis of assessment scales is on observational methods—including assessments of crying patterns, facial expressions, and physiologic parameters (blood pressure, diaphoresis, heart rate, and respiratory rate). Among verbal young children, one can add quantifiable pain assessments (e.g., the "poker chip" tool, "oucher" scale, faces scale). Some instruments (e.g., a visual analog scale and pain diaries) are appropriate for older children and adolescents (Stevens 1997).

The poker chip tool involves use of concrete objects (e.g., poker chips) to quantify or approximate pain ratings. The child is asked to rate the pain intensity by choosing up to four poker chips, depicting "pieces" of hurt. This method can be a particularly useful assessment index for younger children (i.e., ages 4–8 years). One problem with this assessment tool is that the child is unlikely to tease out how much "hurt" is related to pain per se and how much is ascribable to the affective components (e.g., fear associated with the pain).

The oucher scale is a variant of the faces scale, with six photographs of children's expressions in varying degrees of distress organized vertically alongside a numeric scale ranging from 0 to 100. The ratings, however, can vary depending on which anchors are employed. For example, if the lowest pain rating is depicted with a smiling face as opposed to a photograph with a neutral facial expression, different pain ratings might be endorsed. Thus, the examiner is cautioned to use the same scale consistently when comparing pain ratings of a young child over time. There might be differences in pain ratings depending on the ethnic backgrounds and genders depicted in the photographs in the scale as well.

The faces scale (see also Chapter 3, "Evaluation of the Pain Patient," of this book) may be used with children to rate pain severity. The scale is fairly easily understood at about age 6 years and thereafter. It allows one to bypass the potential gender and ethnic biases that can confound pain ratings encountered with the oucher scale.

Pain diaries may be useful for adolescents with pain. Younger children would be expected to be incapable of completing a pain diary, but parents might find such diaries useful. In the diary, pain ratings are ranked and descriptions can be noted of ongoing environmental factors, extenuating circumstances, prevailing mood states, thought patterns, and other factors. The diary can reveal temporal patterns between pain states and mood, thought processes, and extenuating circumstances surrounding the adolescent's pain. Diaries can be useful in encouraging young adults to develop self-management strategies and can foster increased mastery over one's pain.

Analgesics (as outlined further in Chapter 5, "Pharmacology of Pain," of this book) need to be applied judiciously and dosed according to weight (Leith and Weisman 1997) as well as the tolerability of side effects. Routes of administration need to be selected to provide the least invasiveness and distress in application of the analgesic. Very painful conditions (e.g., sickle cell crisis, moderate to severe postoperative pain) may require opiate analgesics. These should not be withheld because of fears of addiction.

Specialized analgesic techniques used with children include local anesthetics and a eutectic mixture of local anesthetics (see Chapter 5 of this book). Patient-controlled anesthesia (PCA) or anesthesia controlled by the parent can be employed for severe pain states. PCA might be best employed with children who are at least age 6 years (Berde and Masek 1999). The advantage of PCA is that the patient can control the amount of analgesic administered. Parent-controlled analgesia raises the risk that misinterpretation of the child's behaviors can result in too little or too much of an analgesic administered. Other interventions might include physical therapy, occupational therapy, and psychotherapeutic interventions. There is strong evidence suggesting that relaxation techniques and cognitive-behavioral therapy can be quite effective in mitigating chronic pain in children and adolescents (Eccleston et al. 2002).

Geriatric Patients

Elderly persons are prone to multiple medical conditions predisposing them to pain. Estimates suggest that rates of chronic pain among elderly persons are twice those of younger individuals (Crook et al. 1984). The elderly are also likely to experience pain from terminal medical conditions (Cleeland 1998). Among community samples, 20%–50% of older persons reported chronic pain (Crook et al. 1984), whereas among those in long-term-care settings, estimates of chronic pain were substantially higher, approaching 45%–80% (Ferrell 1990; Roy and Thomas 1986; Won et al. 1999). Untreated pain interferes with adaptive functioning, interpersonal functioning, and quality of life. Common disorders contributing to chronic pain include arthritis, cancer, diabetic neuropathy, herpes zoster, and osteoporosis (Ferrell 1991; Gallagher et al. 2000).

Underrecognition of Pain in Elderly Patients

Pain is often poorly recognized and poorly treated among the elderly (Sengstaken and King 1993). Reasons include poor recognition of symptoms, inadequate time spent evaluating patients, and failure to inquire about pain symptoms. Appetite and sleep disturbances, social withdrawal, reduced inclination to engage in activities, and distress resulting from pain may be mislabeled as an emotional disturbance (e.g., depression, anxiety). Ascertaining pain may be further hindered by dementia. Inadequate trials of medications to relieve pain, concerns regarding medication's adverse effects, and addiction fears interfere with effective treatment.

Misconceptions that pain sensitivity is reduced among the elderly may be attributed to the unusually painless presentation of some elderly patients with common illnesses. Much has yet to be learned about age-related physiologic changes within the nociceptive pathway system. Although transmission via Aδ and C neurons might be altered with age, the role such changes have in interfering with the recognition or perception of pain remains unclear. Physiologic changes in the nociceptive system occurring with age might not bear much clinical significance (Gagliese et al. 1999).

On the other hand, there might be alterations in the affective (limbic) and cognitive (cortical) processes that are factors in the processing and appreciation of pain. Still, elderly patients could have a reduced inclination to communicate or report pain, which might emanate from belief systems held by some elderly persons (e.g., that pain is to be expected as one ages and therefore does not warrant clinical attention). Further investigation is warranted to assess to what extent such factors influence the perception and reporting of pain among the elderly population.

Nonetheless, careful assessment of the older patient is necessary to effectively address and treat pain. Some education of the patient might be required to circumvent the problems of erroneous expectations interfering with the reporting of pain. Some elderly patients could be concerned that notifying physicians of their pain might invoke treatments that are invasive and painful, that could complicate other health conditions, or that might involve hospitalization and, therefore, separation from family and other usual supports.

Standard assessment scales can be employed in an attempt to quantify the degree of discomfort experienced (see Chapter 3 of this book). Some of these might be easier than others for the elderly to use. Thus, for example, a visual analog scale is harder for elderly patients to comprehend and reliably use than are other assessment devices (e.g., numeric rating scales, faces scale, verbal scales) (Herr and Mobily 1993). Among patients with cognitive impairments that limit effective communication of pain and discomfort, it may be necessary to rely on observation of behavioral changes; some helpful parameters are outlined in Table 9–1.

Table 9–1.   Behavior parameters warranting consideration to assess discomfort

Parameter	Signs
Breathing	Labored, loud, gasping, rapid rate, hyperventilation
Vocalizations	Groaning, moaning, muttering, rapid speech
Facial expression	Tearful, sad, troubled, worried, fearful, alarmed, frowning, scowling
Body language	Tense, strained, fidgety, restless, rubbing or guarding of affected body parts, aggression

Source.   Adapted from Warden V, Hurley AC, Volicer L: "Development and Psychometric Evaluation of the Pain Assessment in Advanced Dementia (PAINAD) Scale." *Journal of the American Medical Directors Association* 4:9–15. Copyright 2003, American Medical Directors Association. Used with permission.

From a biopsychosocial perspective, it becomes imperative to understand the psychological and social factors contributing to the patient's plight and pain. Among the elderly, the psychological issues that prevail include concerns over life review and the need to have fulfilled life goals and to have made contributions to the world.

Treatment Strategies

Older patients are often excluded from studies assessing various medication effects in pain reduction. Often, an attempt is made in clinical trials to avoid the influences of other medical conditions or drug interactions with coadministered medications. Thus, for example, most of the literature on employing psychotropic agents in pain mitigation has largely focused on diverse patient populations and not exclusively on the elderly.

The pharmacologic approaches discussed in Chapter 5 of this book are applicable to the geriatric patient with chronic pain. Opiates might be indicated in acute pain, in chronic malignant pain, and in cases of chronic nonmalignant pain. The elderly can be particularly sensitive to the adverse effects of analgesic agents (e.g., sedation, confusion, constipation associated with opiates, gastrointestinal effects associated with nonsteroidal anti-inflammatory drugs [NSAIDs]) (American Geriatrics Society 1998). In some cases, particularly in patients with neuropathic pain and those with psychological factors contributing significantly to pain, a variety of psychotropic medications are available (Leo and

Singh 2002). In general, the approach with the elderly patient is that initial doses should be low and incremental increases should proceed slowly, guided by the diminution of pain, improvement in function, and tolerability of side effects.

Some effects of pain (e.g., sleep disturbances, appetite suppression) arising from ongoing pain might require attention. Hence, efforts should be directed at the development of sleep hygiene strategies and the selective use of sedating agents (i.e., eszopiclone, zolpidem, zaleplon, trazodone, and possibly benzo-diazepines). Cyproheptadine and megestrol acetate have been employed in situations in which a pharmacologic intervention is selected to increase appetite.

Nonpharmacologic approaches ought to be considered in the treatment of the elderly patient with pain (American Geriatrics Society 1998). These endeavors—including exercise, transcutaneous electrical nerve stimulation (TENS), acupuncture, massage, relaxation training, and psychotherapy, among others—can supplement pharmacologic and other invasive treatment strategies.

Pregnancy

Because of concerns about fetal effects, the use of analgesics during pregnancy has been restricted. Opioid treatment during pregnancy has been documented in cases of women treated with methadone for opiate dependence and with brief opioid requirements during labor. In such cases, the risks to the fetus are outweighed by the potential risks arising from either continued heroin use or complications arising in the delivery process. Nonetheless, concerns still arise with regard to the use of analgesics for pregnant women who experience malignant or nonmalignant pain in the course of pregnancy. Long-term exposure of the fetus to opiates is likely to produce the following effects in the newborn: opiate dependence, acute withdrawal after delivery, and growth retardation. Some patients might still be capable of achieving long-term relief of pain with spinal or intrathecal administration of opiates while minimizing the infant's exposure to the opiate (Wen et al. 1996).

Among other analgesics, NSAIDs administered during pregnancy may prolong labor, result in constriction of the ductus arteriosus in the fetus, and produce renal and hematologic abnormalities in the newborn (Ostensen 1998). Other agents (e.g., aspirin) have been invoked to treat complications in late pregnancy (e.g., preeclampsia), although the risks to fetal growth and development have been a concern.

Use of adjuvant agents (e.g., antidepressants, anticonvulsants) carries with it the risks of fetal complications (e.g., neural tube defects), increased spontaneous abortion rates, and anticholinergic effects in the newborn.

For women who are breastfeeding, acetaminophen and ibuprofen appear to be safest among the nonopioid analgesics because of their high protein binding (Ebert 1997). Most opioids are safe for use during lactation, without harm to the breastfeeding infant. The infant's methadone exposure is determined by the maternal dose and time of breastfeeding in relation to when peak drug effects are obtained. Breastfeeding is permitted for women taking methadone at dosages less than 20 mg/day and should occur at least 6–10 hours after the methadone dose is received (Renehan 1989).

Cultural Issues

With clichés such as "no pain, no gain" and slogans such as "tough it out," one can only be impressed with popular notions about pain. Societal attitudes toward pain may evoke reluctance to report pain and fear of stigma associated with pain complaints.

Although there are no racial or ethnic differences in the ability to discriminate pain (Zatzick and Dimsdale 1990), culture influences what meanings persons derive from illness, suffering, and pain. The psychiatrist addressing pain patients must consider the impact cultural influences might have on the pain experience. Thus, in some black communities, Christian religious beliefs have a profound impact on the understanding of pain. In such communities, suffering has a redeeming function, and efforts to avoid pain might constitute a "failure of faith" (Crawley et al. 2000).

Cultural biases and stereotypes might impede effective pain treatment. Racial and ethnic disparities in pain treatment have been observed in emergency settings (Todd et al. 1993) as well as for cancer, postoperative, and low back pain (Bonham 2001). A multicenter study assessing the adequacy of pain management in cancer found that nonwhite patients with metastatic cancer pain were three times more likely to be undermedicated as compared with white cancer patients (Cleeland et al. 1994). Several factors have been identified that may contribute to disparities in the treatment of pain among nonwhite patients (Table 9–2).

Table 9–2. Barriers to pain management in minority patients

Language
Less frequent follow-up care
  Loss to follow-up
  Poor arrangement of follow-up services
  Poor access to follow-up services
Addiction concerns
Unavailability of analgesics in pharmacies in areas in which minorities live
  (e.g., pharmacies may not stock opiates for fear of theft and violence)
Economic disadvantages (e.g., limited resources result in decisions based on
  paying for analgesics versus paying for other necessities)
Inadequate assessment
  Culturally inappropriate pain rating scales
  Basing of pain assessments on the clinician's perception of overt
    pain behaviors

The tendency to be expressive or unemotional about pain can be dictated by a person's ethnic, religious, and familial background. Language and cultural impediments to pain treatment might be overcome through the use of culturally sanctioned pain assessments. Some assessment instruments (e.g., McGill Pain Questionnaire; see Chapter 3 of this book) have been translated into various languages for such purposes.

Economic disparities affecting certain subcultures might preclude medical follow-up with pain management. Patients living in financially disadvantaged areas might not have access to prescribed analgesics; pharmacies in such areas might not stock analgesics because of fears regarding theft.

Although the prevailing cultural norm within the United States and that of the legal system emphasize the importance of a person's autonomy and the primacy of the individual in decision making, this norm is not shared by many other cultural communities. Thus, among other cultures, the primacy of the family may be emphasized in the decision-making process (Kagawa-Singer and Blackhall 2001). While exploring treatment interventions, the clinician may have to consider varying approaches to decision making, factoring in the need to include others in the patient's life in the proposal of potential treatment options.

222 Clinical Manual of Pain Management in Psychiatry

Substance-Dependent and Substance-Abusing Patients

The patient presenting with pain complaints who simultaneously has ongoing substance abuse or dependence (or a prior history of either) can pose significant challenges in terms of treatment options. Although effective pain management should never be withheld because of an abuse or addiction history, effective treatment might require an array of pain-reducing approaches (e.g., use of adjunctive agents, agents with low abuse potential, physical and psychological therapies, and patient participation in a concurrent substance abuse treatment program). General principles for pain management of this group are outlined in Table 9–3 (Prater et al. 2002; Savage 1998; Scimeca et al. 2000).

The patient's detoxification from the substance(s) on which he or she is dependent might be required before the initiation of treatment. An overly aggressive detoxification can be particularly distressing for patients, perhaps resulting in the inclination to abandon treatment/detoxification. In addition, during the course of detoxification, it could be imperative to undertake simultaneous measures to mitigate pain; otherwise, the distress to which the patient is subjected might be too great, and the patient may develop intense fears that his or her pain will be unrecognized and inadequately treated.

Detoxification is required for the patient who is alcohol dependent. In some cases, the substances abused might have appeal as a means of controlling one's psychological distress (e.g., cannabis and benzodiazepine abuse to address underlying anxiety or ineffective coping). Hence, psychological interventions, along with prudent psychopharmacologic interventions for underlying psychiatric disorders, might also be required to effect optimal pain control.

Patients who receive opiates over the long term for treatment of pain may become addicted to the opiates. This issue is one that raises controversy. Some authors suggest that opiate dependence does not accompany appropriate dosing in pain patients (Portenoy and Foley 1986). Nonetheless, the issue can and does arise—that patients who have been treated with analgesics can become dependent on pain medications.

Iatrogenic Drug Dependence

As mentioned earlier, persons may become addicted to medications prescribed by physicians to treat pain (e.g., opioids, benzodiazepines, stimulants).

Table 9–3. Pain management in patients with substance abuse/dependence

Address pain with
  Pharmacologic strategies
    Nonopioid analgesics are encouraged
    If opioids are required,
        Use those that produce less euphoria
        Scheduled doses are preferred over "as needed"
        Long-acting medications are preferred
  Nonpharmacologic therapies
    Physical/occupational therapy
    Heat/cold therapies
    Transcutaneous electrical nerve stimulation
    Relaxation/hypnosis/biofeedback
    Psychotherapy
Allay fears regarding inadequate pain treatment
Address psychiatric comorbidities
  Depression
  Anxiety
  Sleep disorders
Monitor and treat substance withdrawal (e.g., alcohol, benzodiazepine, opiate)
Support measures to achieve/sustain addiction recovery
  Address detoxification and rehabilitation needs for ongoing substance abuse
  Assess adherence with substance abuse treatment programs
    Consider making opioid analgesia contingent on verifiable participation in addiction recovery treatment program
  Assess for signs of relapse
    Periodic, random urine toxicology screens
    Frequent follow-up and monitoring
        Assessment of overall functioning
        Potential for misuse of extended-release formulations (e.g., injecting extended-release medications intended for oral use)
  Enlist family member or other trusted person to assist with dispensing medication
  Consider use of a patient treatment contract (see Chapter 10)

Source. Adapted from Prater CD, Zylstra RG, Miller KE: "Successful Pain Management for the Recovering Addicted Patient." *Primary Care Companion to the Journal of Clinical Psychiatry* 4:125–131, 2002. Copyright 2002, Physicians Postgraduate Press. Used with permission.

This dependence may occur in a variety of ways. The patient might seek out multiple physicians to acquire such medications, or a single physician may be involved. Patients might offer somatic complaints to acquire medications. The prescription of medications might be construed by the patient as a sign of caring and nurturance. The well-meaning physician might be highly esteemed and valued by the patient and as a consequence might placate the patient's requests for additional medications.

The clinician might not anticipate the patient's risk of dependence on the medications. Often, clinicians are so preoccupied with the patient's allegations of pain that they fail to recognize that increasing levels of medications are being requested or that, despite the use of these medications, the patient's functioning does not appear to improve in adaptive areas. This should signal that the medications are not effective or might be being consumed inappropriately by the patient such that the misused medications interfere with the patient's adaptive function and rehabilitation.

In cases of iatrogenic drug dependence, the patient may require careful systematic detoxification from the medications on which he or she has become dependent. The patient's functioning might then improve. Behavioral measures could be required to de-emphasize the focus on somatic complaints. Cognitive-behavioral interventions might be required to address ineffective coping, troublesome cognitive appraisals, and adverse emotions. It is these emotions the patient has been trying to "treat" with the medications prescribed.

There are concerns that long-term use of opiates might actually interfere with pain mitigating processes. A number of cellular mechanisms are being explored to assess mechanisms underlying tolerance to analgesic efficacy (Fishbain et al. 1992; Streltzer 2001). It should be borne in mind that the opiate-dependent patient requires substantially higher opiate doses to effectively manage severe pain conditions.

Patients With Terminal Conditions

Patients with terminal medical conditions who have pain require compassionate care. In addition to pain management, sensitivity to the patient's perceptions of and concerns regarding death is required. Patients with terminal conditions require regular visitation, a fact frequently ignored by physicians, who often focus on correctable disease or might subconsciously view a patient's death as their failure. Visiting, even when a patient avoids discussions about his or her health or prognosis, conveys that the clinician is reliable, dependable, and available should the occasion (and need) arise to discuss more openly important issues that surround a terminal condition.

Patients may require physical contact, appropriate to the context of the situation, to convey support and attentiveness. Attention to the content of what the patient says is necessary, as is answering the patient's questions in an honest and respectful manner. Patients may inquire about the nature of their illnesses and whether they are at terminal stages. By basing their responses on what is known about the nature and course of the illnesses, physicians can be honest without eradicating hope. Building false hopes is discouraged.

Some patients may find such disclosures to be overwhelming, which the physician may assume is a form of denial. However, this assumption can be insulting to the patient and perhaps intrusive, especially if a psychiatric consultant is asked to evaluate the patient about this presumed denial. Respect for the patient's defenses, even denial, may well be required at such times. Aggressively attempting to eradicate this defensive stance may serve only to distance the patient, causing him or her to become more resistant to the clinician's efforts and care. On the other hand, patients may have fears about asking questions or may not know how to begin making inquiries. The physician might inquire of the patient how much it is he or she wishes to know about the current illness, thus facilitating dialogue on the matter.

Physicians also need to be sensitive about the extent to which the patient, family, significant others, and medical staff are aware of the terminal nature of the patient's illness. Every effort should be made to facilitate communication between the patient and family (and significant others) about the prospect of death—but, again, the issue should be gently and respectfully broached, not forced. Reluctance on the part of the physician to openly discuss such matters may come from fear that the family and patient will think the physician has given up on effective care of the patient or from fears of discouraging or upsetting the patient and family. Opening discussion among the patient and the patient's family could help reduce the isolation, loneliness, and even the dehumanizing features that surround death for the patient. Family conflicts can emerge around the time of death. Opening dialogue between family members at such times can relieve their stress and help them begin the work of bereavement. Family meetings may provide an opportunity for refocusing on the issues that matter.

Physicians may be the target of anger from the patient, the family, or both. Taking a defensive stance in such situations should be avoided. The patient and family might need to ventilate their feelings about death and about the meaning of the patient's illness for them. The best strategy might be to articulate the feelings and emotions underlying the anger, such as "This has been such a long illness and a long struggle for everyone. It is impossible to imagine what it feels like to be challenged with the prospect that our life activities are interrupted prematurely, that our dreams will go unfulfilled." or "It probably feels as though I let you down." Such approaches are likely to diffuse the tension of the impending death and are less likely to escalate into a conflict, as could be the case if the physician took a defensive stance. The doctor may be the safest target of anger, especially if unresolved matters in the patient's relationships are too overwhelming to address directly in the final days.

The family and patient may need reassurance that pain will be maximally controlled. The patient and others may be concerned that pain control will make the patient unaware of his or her surroundings or otherwise incapacitated. Modifying the patient's pain-relief regimen according to his or her wishes is desirable, whereas withholding effective pain treatment to appease the family's need to keep the patient alert is not. Family members may need to be reminded that severe pain will likely mitigate the sedating properties of opiates and other analgesics. The family could also need to be reassured that the analgesics will not result in or hasten the patient's death.

Hospice Care

Hospice care is a system of care for patients with terminal conditions and their families. The goals of therapy within hospice care are to provide palliation (i.e., pain management) but not cure and to ensure dignity of care without the encumbrances of life support measures and invasive procedures.

Care for patients is often arranged in the home, an environment that is familiar and often more comfortable for the patient. Access to the patient by family, friends, and customary supports is more feasible when the patient remains at home. Service to the patient is coordinated among family, other members of the patient's usual support system, medical and mental health personnel, clergy, and volunteers.

Generally, the cost of hospice care is far less than that for hospital care. However, higher costs are incurred when hospice care is provided in nursing homes

Table 9–4.   Medicare requirements for hospice care

Physician must certify that the patient's condition is terminal (i.e., the patient's life expectancy is expected to be 6 months or less).

Patient must consent to hospice care in lieu of traditional hospital care.

Hospice care agency must be certified by Medicare in order to accept benefits from the federal government.

or hospitals or when patients are furnished with care in an established hospice setting. Medicare coverage is provided for hospice care; however, there are limitations to the coverage provided (see Table 9–4). Medicare provides a flat amount for hospice services. Thus, funding provided for a patient expected to live no more than 6 months is quite low, but if the patient lives beyond 6 months, the provision of hospice services continues without reimbursement, and the hospice agency incurs a financial loss. As a result, hospice agencies may be reluctant to accept patients whose illnesses are not inclined to result in death within 6 months. Physicians may be inclined to erroneously withhold an offer of hospice care to patients and their families, fearing that the anticipated time until death might exceed 6 months. Therefore, physicians may be offering hospice care to patients too late in the course of the illness.

As more patients utilize hospice services, psychiatric involvement will be ever increasing in hospice care. Many patients develop psychiatric symptoms either as a consequence of the illnesses that prompted their admission or as effects of treatment. Common psychiatric disturbances likely to be encountered include mood disturbances, anxiety, delirium, and dementia. A number of psychiatric interventions and medications can be employed to reduce the deleterious effects of these psychiatric disturbances. Psychiatrists can be particularly influential in ensuring that pain is adequately addressed in hospice patients.

Family members and friends may have emotional difficulties associated with hospice care. These can include a sense of futility, anticipatory bereavement, guilt (i.e., viewing hospice as a "giving up" on the patient or a withholding of necessary care), and despair. Psychiatrists can be helpful in facilitating the family's adjustment to the hospice care transition and in preventing emotional difficulties from impeding connections with the patient that might be required in the time they have remaining. Psychiatrists can help the family recognize that the focus has become one of ensuring improved quality of life for the patient and can help them maximize the time they have available. Issues concerning death and dying may need to be a focus of care for the patient as well as his or her family and other loved ones.

Religious Issues and Spirituality

Issues of spirituality may be encountered when caring for the patient who has a terminal condition. There may be uncertainties and confusion about treatment decisions (e.g., advance directives), particularly if the patient has fears about the moral implications of a particular treatment. Sometimes religious inquiries can arise when there is a conflict with the physician about prognosis, a distrust of the medical system, and/or a rejection of the physician's expertise. Some patients are distressed about the prognosis and therefore hope for some miraculous intervention. After all, when the prognosis is grim, who would not want a miracle? In situations in which there is persistent pain or severe untoward effects of treatment, some patients may be concerned about punishment, guilt, and prior transgressions.

Many physicians feel unskilled or uncomfortable addressing religious or spiritual issues, often bypassing them to focus on somatic concerns, treatment issues, or even the psychological underpinnings of the discussion (Lo et al. 2002). Yet avoidance of these topics may further increase the patient's isolation as he or she struggles with issues pertaining to such matters. This avoidance may inadvertently jeopardize the therapeutic alliance.

Because of the diversity of concerns that can prompt issues of spirituality, careful inquiry by the physician may expose the patient's underlying concerns or fears (see Table 9–5). While respecting the patient's spiritual issues and dilemmas, the clinician should attempt to reflect religious issues back onto the patient—for example, by inquiring, "Why do you ask?" or "I wonder if you have concerns about what to do next?" Open-ended inquiry can lead to discussions of matters that have an impact on treatment and on the doctor–patient relationship. The clinician is cautioned against being drawn into the potential pitfalls of religious and theological arguments, scriptural interpretations, and so forth that can bypass the patient's underlying concerns. It might be also be prudent to elicit the support of others (e.g., clergy and pastoral counselors) when confronted with moral issues.

Table 9–5. Approaches to dealing with spiritual issues

Use open-ended inquiry.
Acknowledge the patient's spiritual concerns.
Empathize with the patient.
Refocus spiritual questions back onto the patient.
Attempt to clarify whether the patient's spiritual dilemmas concern
   Decisions about further treatment interventions.
   Decisions about advance directives.
   The doctor–patient relationship.
   Questions about the validity and utility of medical interventions.
Avoid reassuring the patient prematurely.
Avoid trying to solve the patient's spiritual dilemmas for him or her.

Key Points

- Pain management approaches need to include psychological, cognitive, and emotional factors pertinent to the needs of patients.
- It is imperative to attend to the unique issues pertinent to the assessment and treatment of pain in special populations, reflective of the patient's cultural norms, age, and stage of development.
- Patients with the greatest barriers to adequate pain treatment include those with known or suspected substance abuse and/or dependence. Such patients are at risk for undertreatment, particularly as clinicians may be fearful of contributing to abuse and addiction.
- Pain management among individuals with abuse and addiction histories requires relatively close monitoring, careful documentation of treatment measures undertaken and outcomes, use of pain treatment contracts, careful utilization of analgesics, and use of adjuvant agents and multimodal treatments to reduce sole reliance on potentially addicting analgesic agents.

References

American Geriatrics Society: The management of chronic pain in older persons: AGS Panel on Chronic Pain in Older Persons. J Am Geriatr Soc 46:635–651, 1998
Berde CB, Masek B: Pain in children, in Textbook of Pain, 4th Edition. Edited by Wall PD, Melzack R. London, England, Churchill Livingstone, 1999, pp 1463–1477

Beyer J, DeGood DE, Ashley LC, et al: Patterns of postoperative analgesic use with adults and children following cardiac surgery. Pain 17:71–81, 1983

Bonham VL: Race, ethnicity, and pain treatment: striving to understand the causes and solutions to the disparities in pain treatment. J Law Med Ethics 29:52–68, 2001

Cleeland CS: Undertreatment of cancer pain in elderly patients. JAMA 279:1914–1915, 1998

Cleeland CS, Gonin R, Hatfield AK, et al: Pain and its treatment in outpatients with metastatic cancer. N Engl J Med 330:592–596, 1994

Crawley L, Payne R, Bolden J, et al: Palliative and end-of-life care in the African American community. JAMA 284:2518–2521, 2000

Crook J, Rideout E, Browne G: The prevalence of pain complaints in a general population. Pain 18:299–314, 1984

Ebert AM: Use of nonnarcotic analgesics during breastfeeding. J Hum Lact 13:61–64, 1997

Eccleston C, Morley S, Williams A, et al: Systematic review of randomised controlled trials of psychological therapy for chronic pain in children and adolescents, with a subset meta-analysis of pain relief. Pain 99:157–165, 2002

Ferrell BA: Pain in the nursing home. J Am Geriatr Soc 38:409–414, 1990

Ferrell BA: Pain management in elderly people. J Am Geriatr Soc 39:64–73, 1991

Fishbain DA, Rosomoff HL, Rosomoff RS: Drug abuse, dependence, and addiction in chronic pain patients. Clin J Pain 8:77–85, 1992

Gagliese L, Katz J, Melzack R: Pain in the elderly, in Textbook of Pain, 4th Edition. Edited by Wall PD, Melzack R. London, England, Churchill Livingstone, 1999, pp 991–1006

Gallagher RM, Verma S, Mossey J: Chronic pain: sources of late-life pain and risk factors for disability. Geriatrics 55:40–47, 2000

Goldschneider KR, Mancuso TJ, Berde CB: Pain and its management in children, in Bonica's Management of Pain, 3rd Edition. Edited by Loeser JD, Butler SH, Chapman CR, et al. Philadelphia, PA, Lippincott Williams & Wilkins, 2001, pp 797–812

Herr KA, Mobily PR: Comparison of selected pain assessment tools for use with the elderly. Appl Nurs Res 6:39–46, 1993

Kagawa-Singer M, Blackhall LJ: Negotiating cross-cultural issues at the end of life: "You got to go where he lives." JAMA 286:2993–3001, 2001

Leith PJ, Weisman SJ: Pharmacologic interventions for pain management in children. Child Adolesc Psychiatr Clin N Am 6:797–815, 1997

Leo RJ, Singh A: Pain management in the elderly: use of psychopharmacologic agents. Annals of Long-Term Care: Clinical Care and Aging 10:37–45, 2002

Lo B, Ruston D, Kates LW, et al: Discussing religious and spiritual issues at the end of life. JAMA 287:749–754, 2002

Ostensen M: Nonsteroidal anti-inflammatory drugs during pregnancy. Scand J Rheumatol 107:128–132, 1998

Portenoy RK, Foley KM: Chronic use of opioid analgesics in non-malignant pain: report of 38 cases. Pain 25:171–186, 1986

Prater CD, Zylstra RG, Miller KE: Successful pain management for the recovering addicted patient. Prim Care Companion J Clin Psychiatry 4:125–131, 2002

Renehan BW: The galactopharmacopedia. Narcotic analgesics: use in the breastfeeding woman. J Hum Lact 5:135–137, 1989

Roy R, Thomas M: A survey of chronic pain in an elderly population. Can Fam Physician 32:513–516, 1986

Savage S: Principles of pain treatment in the addicted patient, in Principles of Addiction Medicine, 2nd Edition. Edited by Graham AW, Schultz TK, Wilford BB. Chevy Chase, MD, American Society of Addiction Medicine, 1998, pp 919–944

Scimeca MM, Savage SR, Portenoy R, et al: Treatment of pain in methadone-maintained patients. Mt Sinai J Med 67:412–422, 2000

Sengstaken EA, King SA: The problems of pain and its detection among geriatric nursing home residents. J Am Geriatr Soc 41:541–544, 1993

Sifford LA: Psychiatric assessment of the child with pain. Child Adolesc Psychiatr Clin N Am 6:745–781, 1997

Stevens B: Pain assessment in children: birth through adolescence. Child Adolesc Psychiatr Clin N Am 6:725–743, 1997

Streltzer J: Pain management in the opioid-dependent patient. Curr Psychiatry Rep 3:489–496, 2001

Todd KH, Samaroo N, Hoffman JR: Ethnicity as a risk factor for inadequate emergency department analgesia. JAMA 269:1537–1539, 1993

Warden V, Hurley AC, Volicer L: Development and psychometric evaluation of the Pain Assessment in Advanced Dementia (PAINAD) scale. J Am Med Dir Assoc 4:9–15, 2003

Wen YR, Hou WY, Chen YA, et al: Intrathecal morphine for neuropathic pain in a pregnant cancer patient. J Formos Med Assoc 95:252–254, 1996

Won A, Lapane K, Gambassi G, et al: Correlates and management of nonmalignant pain in the nursing home. J Am Geriatr Soc 47:936–942, 1999

Zatzick DF, Dimsdale JE: Cultural variations in response to painful stimuli. Psychosom Med 52:544–557, 1990

10

Forensic Issues Pertaining to Pain

Litigation and Pain

Concerns naturally arise about the potential role of ongoing litigation and its effect on the experience of pain, the rehabilitation process, and allegations of disability. It is conceivable that the pursuit of litigation could have an impact on the treatment and rehabilitation of a patient's pain (Gatchel et al. 1995). It has been reported that people with whiplash injuries who were in the midst of litigation reported more pain than those who were no longer involved in litigation (i.e., whose cases were settled or resolved) (Swartzman et al. 1996). However, there was no statistically significant difference between those who were in the midst of litigation and those who were not with regard to employment status, return to work, and functional adaptation. The clinician is cautioned against making causal assumptions about the role of the litigation in influencing the patient's agenda (Swartzman et al. 1996). It is possible that for some patients, pain is exaggerated so as to increase the magnitude of the monetary gain of a litigation claim. On the other hand, it is possible that the stress of the litigation process leads to marked muscle tension, resulting in accentuation and exaggeration of pain complaints. Alternatively, a third factor (e.g., fears of disability, long-term effects of pain, fears of future limitations in work capacity, fears of unemployment and financial hardship) may lead to the simultaneous accentuation of pain complaints as well as the pursuit of litigation.

Careful attention to the types of concerns the patient has could be highly informative in determining which of these interpretations is operating. Attentive listening can lead to those interventions that allay the patient's fears. One of the biggest concerns that patients have is that their pain complaints might not be well received or might be misinterpreted as a ploy to achieve secondary gains. A clinician's reassurance that the clinician is working with the patient to address his or her pain, to improve functional adaptation, and to reduce disability while improving quality of life can help to alleviate such fears. The clinician may need to discuss openly the issues and concerns that beset the patient so that they no longer concern the patient and so they do not adversely affect the doctor–patient relationship.

In addition, pain management has received increasing legal attention. A physician was found guilty of elder abuse based on the premise that he inadequately treated a patient's pain before the patient's death (Albert 2001). In a similar action, a physician was sanctioned by the Oregon Board of Medical Examiners for negligence (i.e., the failure to meet the standard of care as it related to adequate pain management) (Charatan 1999). As these cases illustrate, external pressures are increasing to ensure that physicians are knowledgeable about effective pain management. Consultation with pain management specialists would be warranted in particularly difficult cases.

Medication Diversion

The issues around medication diversion have acquired increasing media, public, and legal attention, especially as related to pain medications. *Diversion* refers to the misappropriation of prescribed medications, either by physicians or by other persons who acquire medications from treating sources. Opiate analgesics of all sorts and varieties can be diverted for their abuse appeal. In the past, agents such as butorphanol had abuse appeal; lately, concerns about diversion have focused on oxycodone. The controlled-release formulation, when crushed and taken into the body intranasally or intravenously, produces a sensation of euphoria; in some communities its popularity has exceeded that of crack cocaine and heroin (Tough 2001).

From a drug regulatory standpoint, medication diversion is difficult to control, because medications are produced by a legitimate pharmaceutical company, prescribed by doctors, and dispensed, presumably, to legitimate patients. There are neither drug lords with whom to contend nor border patrol issues. Instead, the culprits can include physicians (who, for example, acquire illicit drugs in exchange for prescribing medications with diversion appeal), patients, and others associated with legitimate patients who surreptitiously divert the medications meant for the patient. The Internet has become an increasingly popular source of acquisition of controlled substances as well (Forman et al. 2006). For a nominal fee, one's claims are reviewed by an online "physician," who then arranges for delivery of controlled substances to one through the mail. Again, from a drug regulatory standpoint, these Internet sources are difficult to monitor and control.

Many psychoactive medications can be diverted. Clearly, the opiates are particularly appealing for their euphoric effects, allowing the abuser to avoid the encumbrances and risks associated with intravenous heroin abuse. On the other hand, benzodiazepines, barbiturates, and psychostimulants have also been diverted because of their appeal on the street.

Physicians may possibly be colluding with patients in the diversion process. Physicians might be swept away by patient insinuations that if the physician "really cared about" him or her, the medications would be prescribed. Idealization of the physician who complies with the patient's demands and the physician's need for such idealizations can result in the blurring of boundaries that traps the physician into prescribing medications with diversion appeal. Over-identification with the patient and the propensity to assume the mantle of power and authority to alleviate the patient's distress can lead to inappropriate prescription of such medications. In addition, the physician's inward denial regarding reasonable treatment alternatives can interfere with stopping such endeavors. Thus, for example, despite the ongoing pain and distress reported by the patient, the physician ignores alternative strategies to address pain, instead increasing the doses of the opiates (or other requested medications) to appease the patient. The physician can have difficulty managing the hostile, demanding patient, could be unable to set therapeutic limits, and might fear the patient's threats to stop treatment—all of which can perpetuate inappropriate prescribing practices and potential drug diversion.

If diversion is suspected, the physician is entitled to shore up reasonable precautionary practices. Thus, a patient treatment contract (as described below) might be required. The details of the contract can specify that the patient will have to comply with random checks of pill counts to continue in treatment. Exhausting one's prescribed medications shortly after receiving them could suggest that the medications are being diverted to others. The patient might need to be approached to clarify the reasons for the significantly lower than expected pill counts and the whereabouts of that medication. If the drug is insufficiently accounted for, a decision can be made to terminate the treatment plan.

Undertaking legal measures once diversion is substantiated is a consideration, but the clinician faces a risk of confidentiality breach under such circumstances. Legal consultation should be sought before any law enforcement reports are filed. Consultation with colleagues and use of alternative treatment strategies (e.g., use of medications with less abuse or diversion appeal, acupuncture, transcutaneous electrical nerve stimulation units, physical or occupational therapies, massage) could be considered in managing any ongoing pain.

Opiate Adulteration and Misuse

Using an opiate in a manner that is unintended contributes to the abuse potential of such agents and has increased the appeal of diversion of prescribed medications (e.g., the aforementioned ingestion of crushed controlled-release oxycodone for its euphoric effects). It was earlier thought that by antagonizing μ-receptors, less abuse liability would be associated with the opioid agonist-antagonists. Unfortunately, these expectations were not borne out. Thus, it was discovered that some persons pulverize the medication pentazocine and inject it intravenously for its euphoric effects. To counter this, the manufacturer has added naloxone (an opiate antagonist) to the tablet. When taken orally, as intended, the naloxone is poorly absorbed and, therefore, does not interfere with the intended analgesic effects. However, if pulverized and injected, the naloxone becomes fully effective and mitigates any euphoric effect produced by the abuse of this medication. The same approach has been employed to reduce misuse (i.e., intravenous injection) of Suboxone (buprenorphine with naloxone). Butorphanol has been made available as a nasal spray formulation to facilitate ease of administration, particularly in patients with difficulty swallowing. When combined with inhaled antihistamines, butorphanol can produce a euphoric effect similar to that of heroin.

Concerted efforts on the part of clinicians in screening patients for problematic prescription and illicit substance use (e.g., Prescription Drug Use Questionnaire) (Compton et al. 1998) may help to avoid contributing to analgesic misuse and adulteration. In addition, ongoing efforts on the part of the pharmaceutical industry will be necessary to refine strategies that reduce opportunities for adulteration and misuse.

Legal Issues Related to Opioid Prescribing

The federal guidelines for prescribing opioids are defined in the Code of Federal Regulations (CFR), Controlled Substances Act (21, USC 802). An excerpt pertaining to the guidelines for clinicians is provided below:

> A prescription for a controlled substance to be effective must be issued for a legitimate medical purpose by an individual practitioner acting in the usual course of his professional practice. The responsibility for the proper prescribing and dispensing of controlled substances is upon the prescribing practitioner, but a corresponding responsibility rests with the pharmacist who fills the prescription. An order purporting to be a prescription issued not in the usual course of professional treatment or in legitimate and authorized research is not a prescription and the person knowingly filling such a purported prescription, as well as the person issuing it, shall be subject to the penalties provided for violations of the law. (Title 21, CFR 8, 1306.04[a])

The purpose of the Controlled Substances Act is to impart that clinicians, pharmacists, and the patient share responsibilities regarding the regulation of controlled substances. Thus, for the clinician, Schedule II substances should be prescribed only in the context of an ongoing clinician-patient relationship. The clinician should be comfortable that the patient is indeed capable of utilizing the prescribed substances responsibly and that there is a verifiable medical condition that warrants implementing such treatments. Establishing the veracity of the medical condition necessitates a careful history, patient assessment and physical examination, review of medical records, appropriate laboratory investigation, and patient follow-up. Patient monitoring is essential to corroborate responsible use of the prescribed agents and to establish the efficacy of the prescribed agents in terms of pain relief, improvement of adaptive functioning, and overall well-being. There should be a corresponding documentation in the medical record of the above matters, with regular follow-up of patterns of use, efficacy (as suggested by pain scale ratings and functional assessments), any issues pertaining to substance abuse concerns, and justification of continued prescribing of controlled substances, if continued prescribing is necessary.

Pharmacists, likewise, are responsible to ensure that the prescriptions are legitimate, to determine the purpose of the medication, and to verify that the person to whom the medication is dispensed is the intended recipient. If another is acting on behalf of the patient, it may be prudent to ensure that the individual is indeed acting as the patient's representative and to secure government issued photo identification (included in the patient's record). Such measures may mitigate concerns regarding lost or stolen prescriptions.

It is important to recognize that patients are entrusted with the prescribed medications and are likewise imbued with responsibilities according to the CFR. The patient should be apprised that he or she is not to share controlled medications with others, that medications are to be kept locked up in a secure setting, and that if medications are used up prematurely (e.g., using more than 20% of the medication early), the patient must contact the physician to discuss adjustment of the dosing regimen so as to anticipate future prescription needs. In this way, concerns around securing emergency refills and additional medications before the next scheduled visit for the clinician and pharmacist can be allayed and addressed in the treatment relationship.

Patient Contracts

Clinicians may be uncomfortable about prescribing opioids (or other controlled substances) for the long term, especially in chronic nonmalignant pain. The discomfort is often related to concerns about federal regulations, substance abuse, addiction, and diversion. Use of a treatment contract (see Table 10–1) for patients receiving chronic opioid treatment has been advocated by medical and legal experts (Burchman and Pagel 1995), and may help to reinforce adherence with the guidelines offered in the CFR. The contract assumes that the clinician and patient are involved in a mutual endeavor and outlines explicitly the rights and responsibilities of both parties. In this way, both the clinician and the patient are clear about the treatment and are protected on issues pertaining to the use of controlled substances. The contract provides for the appropriate disclosure of these issues and the parameters for treatment—including the use

Table 10–1. Items to be factored into a patient contract for use with controlled substances

Physician responsibilities

Disclose that the substances prescribed are controlled by local, state, and federal agencies.

Specify that prescriptions for controlled substances will be made only during regular office hours—not at night, on weekends, on holidays, and so forth.

Specify that unknown risks may be associated with long-term use of controlled substances and that the patient will be kept apprised of any advances in the field that call attention to such risks.

Disclose information regarding potential development of tolerance and physical dependence.

Specify the grounds for termination of prescription of controlled substances.

Patient responsibilities

Prevent loss, misplacement, or theft of controlled substances, understanding that controlled substances will not be readily replaced.

Be present in person to pick up prescriptions for controlled substances.

Take the medication in the dose and at the intervals prescribed.

Keep track of the amount of medication remaining.

Comply with random urine or blood testing to document the proper use of medications and confirm adherence.

Comply with the laws of the state regarding use of medications and operation of motorized vehicles.

Work with the physician in developing better health habits.

Do not divert or dispense controlled substances to others.

---

and acquisition of analgesics and other treatment responsibilities. The patient is made aware of his or her responsibilities with regard to use of the medication; other responsibilities regarding participation in nonpharmacologic facets of treatment (e.g., physical therapy, smoking cessation, avoidance of alcohol, weight loss, psychotherapy, substance abuse treatment) can also be delineated. The patient is informed that violation of the conditions of the contract can allow the physician to terminate the use of controlled substances. The contract can specify limitations regarding the acquisition of controlled substances (e.g., that prescriptions will not be provided for "running out early," prescription loss, or spilled or misplaced medications) and can state that prescriptions should not be acquired from other clinicians, emergency departments, or after-hours facilities. A copy of the contract, signed by the clinician and the patient, can be given to the patient; the original should be filed in the patient's chart. In this way, the contract can serve as a basis for the overall treatment plan.

Drug Testing in Clinical Practice

Drug testing is increasingly utilized in the clinical setting, particularly because it can assist with complex medical and legal aspects of pain management care. Although drug testing can create a level of discomfort for clinician and patient alike, recommendations for urine drug testing may offer several advantages to the care of patients, especially those with chronic, nonmalignant pain, requiring long-term opioids and other controlled substances for pain relief (Heit and Gourlay 2004). (Some of these advantages are outlined in Table 10–2.) It should be recognized that with open disclosure and dialogue regarding the uses of drug testing within the scope of the clinician–patient treatment relationship, some of the discomfort associated with the stigma of drug testing can be allayed. It is imperative, however, that appropriate documentation and diagnostic information be provided to ensure accuracy of the testing and appropriately secure patient confidentiality. Clinicians also need to be aware that there are several mechanisms by which individuals can attempt to undermine testing. These can include provision of substitute urine from another person, adulteration of the urine sample so as to conceal substances, and dilution of the sample, necessitating that certain standardized procedural measures be implemented in securing that samples are appropriately obtained and handled for testing. On the other hand, the advantage of urine testing can be a factor that leads to the development of mutual trust between clinician and patient, bolstering the therapeutic alliance.

State and National Prescribing Data Banks

Because of concerns regarding abuse and diversion of prescription medications, President Bush signed the National All Schedules Prescription Electronic Reporting Act into law on August 11, 2005. It is hoped that sweeping changes will occur across the country as a result, such that by 2010 all states will have to establish drug monitoring programs. The purpose of the moni-

Table 10–2. Advantages of urine drug testing in clinical pain management practice

Urine drug testing provides

A baseline identification of drug use on admission

Corroboration of prescription drug adherence

Identification of medications provided by other treatment providers and verification of patient's history

Identification of other disease states that can complicate treatment planning (e.g., kidney disease, diabetes)[a]

Identification of illicit substance use

Confirmation of or refuting of concerning behaviors manifested by the patient (e.g., intoxicated appearances, pill count discrepancies, requests for early refills)

Delineation of the need for substance abuse treatment

A barrier to diverting controlled substances

Proof of complying with federal regulatory standards that the clinician is monitoring controlled substances prescribed

An objective therapeutic regimen for reports to insurance providers, workers' compensation, medical boards, and other regulatory agencies

Reduced mistrust on the part of the clinician regarding the patient's presentation and behavior

---

[a]When combined with macroscopic urinalysis.
Source. Adapted from Fornari FA, Siwicki DM, Bauer GB: "Urine Drug Testing and Monitoring in Pain Management." *Practical Pain Management* 6:12–14, 2006. Copyright 2006, PPM Communications. Used with permission.

toring program is to establish a data bank that allows physicians and pharmacists to access patient records, track the prescription of controlled substances, and avoid duplicate prescribing of controlled substances. (The purposes of the database system are outlined in Table 10–3.)

Additionally, clinicians will be held accountable for updating such systems and tracking medications prescribed by other treating sources through the data bank. In this way, the clinicians will be expected to review the controlled substances that have already been prescribed, avoid overprescribing, and monitor for potential untoward reactions and drug interactions. Unfortunately, such measures can impose a greater burden on clinicians with regard to tracking patient treatment. Further, there may be greater liability for clinicians for

Table 10–3. Purposes of the National All Schedules Prescription Electronic Reporting Act database system

As a national database, allows for the tracking of

Patient prescription use

Prescribing patterns of medical practitioners

Prescribing patterns according to geographical regions

Prescribing rates and patterns of controlled medications

As a clinician access database, allows for the

Tracking of your patient's prescriptions

Assessment and evaluation of efficacy of prior and current medications prescribed

Continuous appraisal of medications prescribed to the patient by other treatment providers

Ascertainment of whether controlled substances are obtained from multiple providers and pharmacies concurrently

Monitoring for the potential of drug interactions

untoward effects from prescribing, especially when the information in the data bank will be at one's disposal.

Naturally, with such a system, it is possible to access information about what medications the patient has been prescribed, by whom, and why. Concerns over issues regarding confidentiality are likely to be raised from such endeavors. Nonetheless, when the system is fully implemented, and several states have already begun to initiate such data bank efforts, patients may need to be apprised of the disclosure of such information, its accessibility, and implications for their care.

Confidentiality

Patient information can be released only with the authorization of the patient or under proper legal compulsion. For the release authorization to be valid, the patient must be informed of the purposes of the release and of the recipient(s) to whom the information will be sent. At times, the patient must be informed of the extent of the information released and its contents. Of course, to authorize release of information, the patient must be competent to give consent for the release (American Psychiatric Association Committee on Confidentiality 1987).

Clinicians must always ensure that the contents of the patient's medical record are kept confidential. In the era of managed care and the sweeping demands of insurance companies, reimbursement is often tied to the review of the medical record (Hartmann 2001). Physicians often find that their business interests (e.g., reimbursement) are at odds with patient protection. Patients need to be apprised that the contents of the medical record might be requested for reimbursement to be possible. If request for this information is refused, the insurance company might not make payments for the cost of the services provided. It may be possible in some cases to withhold, without adversely influencing reimbursement, selected aspects of the record that the patient finds too difficult to divulge.

In addition, relevant, easily identifiable information pertaining to a specific patient's case cannot be divulged for educational, training, or publication purposes. If the content of a patient's history, presentation, or similar information is to be used for such purposes, every effort should be made to remove any identifying information that would allow the intended audience to identify the source.

The courts might require that physicians divulge the confidential information contained in a medical record. Legal consultation might be required to assist the clinician in determining the extent of the information that needs to be disclosed. At times, the full content of the record is not required, and particularly personal matters might be best avoided in the legal forum to protect the patient's privacy.

To protect a patient (or another person) from imminent danger, it might be required that the clinician reveal confidential information (*Tarasoff v. Regents of the University of California* 1976). Thus, if a patient threatens self-harm, has a realistic plan, is at risk for lethality, and is not working with the clinician in any way to ensure his or her safety, the clinician might have no recourse but to divulge aspects of the history to potential sources of help who might be able to mobilize the patient's safety (e.g., family, friends, police, crisis services). The clinician must have good cause to suspect that the patient (or another person) is at risk of imminent danger and that other alternatives are not available to remediate the situation. Again, the extent of the information revealed could be limited to only those aspects that will affect the decision making at hand and ensure the safety of the patient and others. Clinicians must be familiar with state laws that regulate such disclosures and with limitations of the confidentiality regulations.

Disability Compensation

Disability Versus Impairment

A *disability* is a putative deficit in functioning, implying a lack of ability to perform activities required for work. It is rather subjective (i.e., is a perception of restriction of function). On the other hand, an *impairment* is an abnormality in psychological or physiologic functioning, verifiable by a clinician and based on observable findings (e.g., physical and mental status examination, laboratory findings). The determination of eligibility for disability awards can be quite complex, and the standards vary depending on the agency from which the award is sought. The basis for the claim involves a review of evidence gathered from a number of medical and, in some cases, nonmedical sources.

Workers' Compensation

Workers' compensation is a system of laws ensuring that compensation awards are provided for persons who sustain injuries during the course of work; it does not litigate fault or negligence (Crook 1994). The goal of workers' compensation is to provide injured employees with money to cover the costs of medical expenses and provide some portion of lost wages. A person who is injured while on duty is not entitled to intangible compensation (e.g., for pain and suffering). Critical to the award is the nature of the alleged injury and its relationship to the work setting. A compensable physical or mental injury must be reasonably connected to the work. The injury cannot arise solely from the worker's own health risks (e.g., coronary artery disease brought on by years of cigarette smoking). Similarly, preexisting illnesses are not compensable. However, preexisting illnesses can predispose a person to complications arising from work injuries. In such cases, the injury and its treatment are compensable. To qualify as compensable, the injury must be accidental and cannot be deliberately self-inflicted.

Critical to workers' compensation is the establishment that the impairment interferes with the performance of prior work. *Prior work* includes those jobs that are suitable to, or related to, one's training and qualifications. Determinations of awards are contingent on the anticipated prognosis and the impact of the injury on one's functional capacity. *Functional capacity* refers to one's abilities to perform activities of daily living, manage one's finances, maintain relationships, and so forth.

Table 10–4.   Limitations considered by Social Security Administration adjudicators

Physical limitations	Mental limitations
Exertional	Understanding and memory deficits
Postural	Concentration deficits
Manipulative	Deficits in social interaction
Visual	Deficits in adaptation
Communicative	Severe emotional disturbances
Environmental	Psychosis

Social Security Disability

Unlike workers' compensation awards, Social Security disability awards are based on the finding that one's physical or mental impairment interferes with the ability to perform any job in the national economy, not just one's former job (see Table 10–4).

The impairment cannot be transient but must be present for a continuous period of at least 12 months (Social Security Administration 2001). According to the Social Security Administration (SSA), to be eligible for disability the impairment must preclude working to meet a minimum standard of financial income. Essential to the assessment of claims of pain disabilities is the assessment of one's functional capacity (Enelow and Leo 2002) (including activities of daily living and ability to lift, carry, push, pull, sit, stand, walk, manipulate, see, hear, understand, remember, concentrate, and follow simple instructions). In addition to financial compensation, recipients can become eligible for medical insurance (i.e., Medicaid or Medicare) (Institute of Medicine 1987; Leo and Del Regno 2002).

Veterans Affairs Benefits

The U.S. Department of Veterans Affairs (VA) offers a disability program for disabled American veterans. Unlike the SSA, no means test is required, and unlike the SSA and workers' compensation systems, there is no requirement that the individual demonstrate an inability to work. Compensation through the VA is of two types: service-connected benefits (i.e., for disabilities acquired in the course of military service) and non-service-connected benefits (i.e., for disabilities acquired after military service and precluding ability to work at a substantial level) (Institute of Medicine 1987). In order to be compensable, the alleged mental and/or physical disability must be validated by medical sources and must be expected to last indefinitely. For a person to qualify for benefits, a clinician must provide medical documentation that substantiates the allegation of a disorder that is grounded in anatomic or physiologic evidence and appropriate clinical signs and symptoms. In addition to financial awards, beneficiaries are eligible to receive medical care provided through the VA health system, including physical rehabilitation, prosthetic devices (if required), and vocational rehabilitation services.

Disability and the Doctor–Patient Relationship

Several issues need to be addressed with the patient who intends to file a claim for disability benefits (Mischoulon 2002), because the outcome of the disability determination can have an impact on the doctor–patient relationship. Ambivalence may arise in response to a favorable decision. Although allowance of a disability award means access to resources of financial support and medical insurance, it might also stir up feelings of dependency, inadequacy, and loss of self-sufficiency in the patient. On the other hand, an unfavorable decision might be interpreted negatively (e.g., a withholding of needed resources). Such feelings can be directed at the treating physician. Discussions between the physician and patient before the claim is submitted could possibly diffuse these potential reactions and prevent them from impeding the treatment alliance.

It would be prudent for the physician to review with the patient the process by which disability determinations are made, emphasizing that the physician does not make the decision about disability eligibility but that the decision rests with adjudicators (and possibly judges and courts if appeals are undertaken). In addition, patients should be apprised that the physician is but one source contacted by disability adjudicators for clinical information and that clinical information is considered in light of information provided from other sources.

It is imperative that a signed release of information be obtained before any information is disclosed to any agency determining disability eligibility. The limits of confidentiality need to be disclosed to the patient (American Psychiatric Association Committee on Confidentiality 1987). Addressing this matter directly avoids the potential for confrontations regarding disclosure of sensitive information after it has been provided to disability or compensation reviewers.

The nature of the disability program intrinsically creates incentives for claimants to maximize monetary gains by emphasizing functional limitations and overstating the severity of illnesses (Fontana and Rosenheck 1998). The person with mild symptoms who dramatizes the severity of his or her disability can trigger marked countertransference reactions in the clinician (Heiman and Shanfield 1978). Physicians might harbor resentment and other feelings at being pulled into the position of rewarding idleness, inactivity, and dependency. Inattention to countertransference reactions can lead the physician to underestimate the severity of the claimant's symptoms, distance himself or herself from the patient, and thereby undermine any attempts at rehabilitation.

Clinicians could have concerns about the unstructured time patients have once disability benefits are awarded. There could be concerns that treatment endeavors (e.g., development of autonomy and self-sufficiency) might be undermined. Among the factors that adversely influence return to work after a disabling injury is the length of time spent on disability compensation (Chatfield 1998). Other factors include current litigation, significant depression and psychiatric comorbidity, substance abuse, and lack of personal satisfaction with work (Chatfield 1998).

Directly addressing such concerns with the patient could be meaningful and therapeutic (i.e., laying the foundation for vocational rehabilitation and work preparatory skills). In addition, the time available off work might allow for pursuit of more intensive treatment, including psychotherapy, group therapy, and day treatment. In this way, the pursuit of disability benefits does not become an end in itself but a means to improve the rehabilitation of the patient.

Key Points

- Ongoing litigation issues and pursuit of disability claims may contribute to the experience of pain (e.g., predisposing patients to exaggeration of perceived disability and reinforcing patients' overt pain behaviors).
- Increasingly, legal action has been undertaken on behalf of patients for whom pain has been inadequately treated. Such trends reflect the societal standards regarding the importance of pain management and the premium placed on having clinicians in virtually all medical specialties appropriately trained in pain management treatment strategies.

- Preventing drug abuse is an important societal concern. Standards put forth by the Code of Federal Regulations attempt to codify responsibilities of all parties involved in the prescription, dispensing, and use of analgesics and potentially addicting medications. Additional measures (e.g., the National All Schedules Prescription Electronic Reporting Act) are being implemented in order to reduce the likelihood of inordinate prescription of controlled substances and to minimize the risks of diversion and misappropriation of controlled substances.
- Clinicians are often at the forefront of ensuring that controlled substances are prescribed for legitimate medical purposes. Vigilance for possible adulteration or abuse of such substances, or for controlled substance misappropriation and diversion, is warranted. Regular medical follow-up, documentation of treatment response and functional assessments, periodic pill counts, and judicious use of drug testing in clinical practice may be helpful.
- Use of a treatment contract may be helpful in establishing goals of treatment and stipulating conditions upon which continued treatment will be based.
- Determination of eligibility for disability awards can be complex; the standards vary depending upon the entitlement program from which the award is sought (i.e., workers' compensation, Veterans' Affairs, or Social Security Disability Insurance or Supplemental Security Income). Clinicians need to be cognizant of the potential pitfalls to the doctor–patient relationship that may arise from pursuit of disability claims. Addressing such impediments in the therapeutic context is necessary so as to mitigate potential barriers to rehabilitative and treatment endeavors.

References

Albert T: Doctor guilty of elder abuse for undertreating pain. Am Med News, July 23, 2001, pp 1, 4

American Psychiatric Association Committee on Confidentiality: Guidelines on confidentiality. Am J Psychiatry 144:1522–1526, 1987

Burchman SL, Pagel PS: Implementation of a formal treatment agreement for outpatient management of chronic nonmalignant pain with opioid analgesics. J Pain Symptom Manage 10:556–563, 1995

Charatan F: Doctor disciplined for "grossly undertreating" pain. BMJ 319:728, 1999

Chatfield JW: Symptom magnification: an overview from clinical practice, in Pain Management: A Practical Guide for Clinicians, 5th Edition, Vol 2. Edited by Weiner RS. Boca Raton, FL, St Lucie Press, 1998, pp 737–742

Compton P, Darakjian J, Miotto K: Screening for addiction in patients with chronic pain and "problematic" substance use: evaluation of a pilot assessment tool. J Pain Symptom Manage 16:355–363, 1998

Controlled Substances Act, Title 21, Code of Federal Regulations CFR 8, 1306.04(a), (USC 802)

Crook PL: Worker's compensation, in Handbook of Pain Management, 2nd Edition. Edited by Tollison CD, Satterthwaite JR, Tollison JW. Baltimore, MD, Williams & Wilkins, 1994, pp 722–731

Enelow AJ, Leo RJ: Evaluation of the vocational factors impacting on psychiatric disability. Psychiatr Ann 32:293–297, 2002

Fontana A, Rosenheck R: Effects of compensation-seeking on treatment outcomes among veterans with posttraumatic stress disorder. J Nerv Ment Dis 186:223–230, 1998

Forman RF, Woody GE, McLellan T, et al: The availability of web sites offering to sell opioid medications without prescriptions. Am J Psychiatry 163:1233–1238, 2006

Fornari FA, Siwicki DM, Bauer GB: Urine drug testing and monitoring in pain management. Practical Pain Management 6:12–14, 2006

Gatchel RJ, Polatin PB, Mayer TG: The dominant role of psychosocial risk factors in the development of chronic low back pain disability. Spine 20:2702–2709, 1995

Hartmann L: Confidentiality, in Ethics Primer of the American Psychiatric Association. Edited by the American Psychiatric Association Ethics Committee. Washington, DC, American Psychiatric Association, 2001, pp 39–44

Heiman EM, Shanfield SB: Psychiatric disability assessment: clarification of problems. Compr Psychiatry 19:449–454, 1978

Heit HA, Gourlay DL: Urine drug testing in pain medicine. J Pain Symptom Manage 27:260–267, 2004

Institute of Medicine Committee on Pain, Disability, and Chronic Illness Behavior: Disability determination and the role of pain, in Pain and Disability: Clinical, Behavioral, and Public Policy Perspectives. Edited by Osterweis M, Kleinman A, Mechanic D. Washington, DC, National Academy Press, 1987, pp 37–65

Leo RJ, Del Regno P: Social Security claims of psychiatric disability: elements of case adjudication and the role of primary care physicians. Prim Care Companion J Clin Psychiatry 3:255–262, 2002

Mischoulon D: Potential pitfalls to the therapeutic relationship arising from disability claims. Psychiatr Ann 32:299–302, 2002

Social Security Administration: Disability evaluation under Social Security (SSA Publ No 64–039). Baltimore, MD, Social Security Administration, January 2001

Swartzman LC, Teasell RW, Shapiro AP, et al: The effect of litigation status on adjustment to whiplash injury. Spine 21:53–58, 1996

Tarasoff v Regents of the University of California, 17 Cal 3d 425, 551 P2d 334, 131 Cal Rptr 14 (1976)

Tough P: The OxyContin underground. The New York Times Magazine, July 29, 2001, pp 50–63

Index

Page numbers printed in **boldface** *type refer to tables or figures.*